LOVE AS HEALING

Documenting a Family's Devoted Emotional Struggle with Functional Movement Disorder (FMD)

Young-hee SHIM and Sang-jin HAN

LOVE AS HEALING
Documenting a Family's Devoted Emotional Struggle
with Functional Movement Disorder (FMD)

Published by Joongmin, LLC., USA, an imprint of
Joongmin Publishers, Seoul, Korea.

Joongmin, LLC.
1212 Luanne Ave, Fullerton, CA 92831, USA

Joongmin Publishers
4th Floor, 20-3, Beobwon-ro 3gil, Seocho-gu, Seoul, 06595, Korea
blog.naver.com/jmpublisher
jmpublisher@naver.com

For information about this title or to order other books
and/or electronic media, contact the publisher:

ISBN: 979-8-9887288-0-1 (softcover)
ISBN: 979-8-9887288-1-8 (ebook)

Printed in the United States of America

Cover and Interior design: 1106 Design

*Dedicated to all FMD sufferers
and their families around the world*

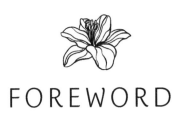

FOREWORD

. . .

"Functional Movement Disorder Syndrome. It's caused by stress."

THIS WAS MY DIAGNOSIS, THE name of my illness. The illness brought terrible symptoms. I experienced flare ups, again and again, in which lumps of muscle on my body jerked from side to side, and at times my entire body shook as if it were shivering from cold. I didn't know what kind of illness I was suffering from, or which hospital or department I needed to go to for treatment. I looked around everywhere, and finally found a neurologist who gave me a confirmable diagnosis.

Diagnosed in precise academic terms as experiencing 'functional' or 'psychogenic' movement disorder syndrome, I underwent a brain MRA, a spinal MRI, a brain wave scan, and an electromyogram. Then, as my condition spiraled, I underwent all sorts of other tests, including the Huntington genetic test and an autoimmunity test. The test results showed only normal values, no abnormalities. Yet I continued to experience brutal and uncontrollable tremors.

"Psychogenic" disease is a vague term. Only recently has a specific name for the disease, 'movement disorder syndrome', been discussed. 'Psychogenic' means that the disease is *of the mind*, and as one doctor told me, it's probably rooted in stress. The symptoms are similar to Parkinson's disease and hand tremors, but the specifics of its diagnosis and treatment are still unclear. Because little is known about the disease, there aren't many studies about it, and there is no specific treatment for it.

My own symptoms of 'movement disorder syndrome' began to appear in the spring of 2019. The first doctor who checked my symptoms looked at my brain MRA results and told me not to worry as there was no serious problem. However, as the symptoms worsened, my neck and back began to pulsate violently, and my muscles repeatedly tensed and contracted. My whole body was in spasms and I couldn't sleep, and when I couldn't sleep, my condition worsened the next day, and I stayed in bed, unwilling to get up. This created a vicious cycle of worsening symptoms.

My husband, in an attempt to do something to break the cycle, encouraged me to get out of the house and exercise, saying that I needed to walk to regain my energy. In order to walk, someone had to support my arm, which throbbed spasmodically. Eventually, as the symptoms worsened, my right arm stayed stuck down at my side and I couldn't lift it. The muscles in my back moved irregularly too, making it impossible to walk normally. In addition, I suffered paralysis in my fingers and was unable to use my hands.

I couldn't speak well, I couldn't eat properly, and even drinking water was a challenge. I couldn't do anything without someone's help. When I couldn't breathe freely because my lungs were giving me trouble, I cried a lot, wondering "What sin did I commit to deserve this?" I even wished my life would end so that I wouldn't have to suffer anymore.

Because I'd always enjoyed good health, my family was distraught at my sudden debility. While my husband and children were looking into various methods of treatment, I mulled over what kind of stress could have caused my illness. At some point, there must have been some big shock, or perhaps multiple incidences of anxiety that had accumulated over a long period and caused my body to convulse in repetitive involuntary tensing and contracting movements.

The doctor said that the cause was stress. I doubt I'd ever even thought about how I handled stressful situations, as I'd always kept my focus forward as I ran through life. During periods of extreme stress, I endured things alone and didn't discuss them openly.

One can only speculate as to the type of stress I experienced and how intense it was in order for me to get this illness. Neither the medical staff nor I myself can ever know exactly what made me ill. It was, after all, more important to release the stress than try to figure out where it came from. My belief now is that relieving stress requires one to have the courage to talk to someone about it, to ask for help as soon as possible, rather than endure it alone.

This book is a record of the pain and suffering caused by the disease called 'functional movement disorder syndrome', how I gradually got out of that pain, and, in particular, how important the help of my family was to my recovery. During the worst part of my illness, my hands were paralyzed and I couldn't even move them, much less write. When things got better, I tried to write again, but I couldn't remember certain events well, so I looked over the notes I'd written on the calendar, and at the photos and videos my family took at that time, to jog my memory. My husband's meticulous records that he kept all throughout the caregiving process proved to be a most reliable and important source of data for this book.

The first and third parts of this book were written by me, and the second part by my husband. Part 1 of the book deals with the onset of my illness when I first endured symptoms such as tremors, stiffness, and paralysis. Part 2 was written by my husband, who cared for and helped me during the most difficult period from July through September 2019. It's a compilation of the records he kept at that time. Part 3 covers the recovery process in which I had to seek out alternative means of treatment and ultimately relearn everything from the beginning.

Although I've published many sociology books and papers, this is the first time I've discussed *myself*, and I was initially embarrassed and hesitant to write a work of this kind. Looking back, I felt very confused at first because I didn't know what kind of disease I had or how to deal with it. I also felt deeply concerned that there was so little information available on the topic. I thought that sharing my experiences with others in a similar situation could be of some help.

How to read the book is entirely up to the reader, but as the author, I'd like to add a small guide: Part 1 is about the symptoms, Part 2 is about my family's experiences and responses, and Part 3 is about the healing process, my overcoming of the illness.

My husband hesitated until the very end about becoming a co-author. However, it would have been difficult to complete the book if it hadn't been for the records he kept. I couldn't keep myself grounded without his help, I couldn't use my hands, and I had a lot of trouble sleeping at night. I remember that it was very painful, but not all of the details. What I couldn't recall was recorded in my husband's meticulous notes, which he made every day after I went to sleep and until the wee hours of the morning. These notes became a valuable record that let us feel a sense of unity as a husband and wife again. As my husband's share in the book grew, I persuaded him that it was only a matter of course for him to become a co-author.

When the original Korean language version of this book was published in June 2022, the fourth year of my battle with the disease, one of my physicians, Professor Park Jung E (Neurology Department, Dongguk University's Ilsan Hospital) recommended the publication of an English translation. She was trained for several years on Functional Movement Disorder Syndrome under the guidance of Professor Mark Hallett at the National Institutes of Health in the U.S. So, on the recommendation of Professor Kwon Young-min of the Department of Korean Literature at Seoul National University, I asked Ga Baek-lim to translate my book. He has studied Korean literature for a long time and has translated several Korean works into English. I am deeply grateful for his hard work in translating the book wonderfully in close detail and elegant English.

I'd like to thank my family for taking care of me with great love while we were fighting this disease, my friends who gave me warmth and comfort, and the medical staff, including Professor Jeon Beomseok of Seoul National University Hospital. I'd also like to express my deep gratitude to my care helper Eun-young who unfailingly supported me in my painful physical state. In addition, my gratitude is extended to writer Heo Hyeon-ja, who compiled my personal account and my husband's journal entries into one book and made it easier to read. I'd also like to express my gratitude to Cho Myoung-ok and Choe Myeong-ji at Joongmin Publishers, who have devoted their time to publishing Korean and English version of this book. I'd also like to thank Dr. Peter Moody for his meticulous reading of the translated manuscript; Michelle and Ronda of 1106 Design for the cover and interior design of the English version; and Ingram Spark for the print publication.

Above all, I'd like to express my deepest gratitude, with all the love in the world, to my husband who, suffering from sleep deprivation due to his care-giving when I was very ill, kept detailed daily records so that the things I couldn't remember could be included in this book.

Encouraged by the love and help I received during my illness, the warm support of my families, friends, and caregivers, I wanted to do something, however small, for other FMD patients. Recalling the difficulties we experienced due to lack of the information about the disease, my husband and I started an on-line cafe for FMD patients (https://cafe.naver.com/jmfmd), where FMD patients and their families can help and encourage one another with information-sharing and self-help tips.

Finally, I hope that the message of this book, namely, 'family love is the path to healing', will resonate and be appreciated, not only among Eastern readers but among Western readers, as well.

May 31, 2023
Shim Young-hee

ENDORSEMENTS TO THE ENGLISH EDITION

• • •

Love As Healing is a story of triumph through courage and devotion over a terrifying and poorly understood disease. It has its hero and heroine—two prominent and dynamic Korean sociologists with lifetimes of public dedication behind them, faced suddenly with a sickness which stems from the mind and sets out to paralyse the body. It records their lengthy and laborious search for treatments which worked and shows how they found one together: not "the talking cure", but a long slow cure through love. It is inspiring, humbling, medically illuminating, and as intensely Korean as it is resonantly universal in its message.

John Dunn
Professor Emeritus of Cambridge University, UK

Functional movement disorders have been known since the dawn of medicine, but in the latter part of the 20th century they were neglected. Physicians were not educated about them, and patients were undiagnosed and went from doctor to doctor. This sad situation is now being changed with better education, better understanding with explanation by a biopsychosocial model, and better treatments. This interesting book details the course of the disorder in a highly educated woman and the impact on her family, particularly her husband, who took on the role of caregiver. The detail of the story is unmatched in the literature and shows the difficulties that patients have and the improvements that can be made by taking into account psychological and social factors. What can be better than love?

Mark Hallett
MD, NINDS Scientist Emeritus,
National Institutes of Health, USA

I have known Shim Young-hee and her husband Han Sang-jin for more than 50 years since they began their doctoral studies. *Love As Healing* is a moving account of how a woman accustomed to flying high from one academic venue to another is brought low by a mysterious attack on her body that affected her and her family emotionally. She writes early in the book: "My Life Is Destroyed and My Dreams Vanish." Yet, she tells us of the long struggle to learn even breathing and walking. Today Young-hee is well again, in large part because her family cared for her beyond what physicians could do. Love heals! *Love As Healing* is a book of lessons—not just for the ill seeking recovery—but for all who are torn by wars or civil strife. Above all, it teaches us that we all need either family or family-like friends to survive any illness and, by implication, to live in this troubled world.

Charles Lemert
Professor Emeritus of Wesleyan University, USA

ENDORSEMENTS TO THE KOREAN EDITION

• • •

"Make a boast of your disease", they say. But this isn't so easy, which is why the saying was born. Illness often remains a well-guarded secret. In the past, stealing a monarch's medical prescriptions or health records was a deadly crime. Nowadays, all medical records are strictly confidential under the Privacy Act.

Crafting beautiful prose is a good thing. It's wonderful to shed light on the darkness of the world, to reform it through writing.

In their many writings to date, Shim Young-hee and Han Sang-jin, a married couple, have done an outstanding job of enlightening and seeking to dispel darkness where they find it.

Now, Professor Shim has written a record of her personal struggle with disease, and Professor Han, her life partner, has written about his struggle as a caregiver. Here, the two merged their respective accounts into one book. It is a wonderful thing that they try to help others who suffer from the same disease that they fought. I commend them for that.

Not only is the disease dealt with in this book largely unknown to the general public, it can also be a sensitive subject to discuss.

If parts of your body tremble without your willing it, or if you're unable to move, we suspect an abnormality in the brain. If it turns out to be a brain disorder, that diagnosis is easily accepted. But if no such anomaly is present—if the symptoms point to a functional problem—then it becomes hard to understand how those symptoms might result from something other than free will.

We believe in free will, that all thoughts and deeds are of our own volition. But the nature of the relationship between the brain and the mind, the degree to which free will manifests itself in the brain, is still an unsolved debate in science and philosophy. One thing is clear: what we believe to be our thoughts and will are the result of actions in the brain that we either do not feel or we do not notice.

The concept of functional or psychogenic movement disorders has changed since the time of Charcot, the early French authority in modern neurology. The current medical understanding can be described as follows: *the occurrence of abnormal tremors due to a group of factors which can be generally referred to as stress, with responses that differ from conscious willful action, although there are no structural changes in the brain.*

The illness is diagnosed clinically. A test is conducted to reassure the patient regarding the absence of brain abnormalities. The most important determinant for the success of the treatment is that the patient accepts the diagnosis. As the reader will see in this book, it is difficult to understand that an 'illness of the mind', of which one is not even aware, can lead to the appearance of severe abnormalities. This is natural because we believe in personal free will. But sometimes our minds are fragile, and sometimes we need the help of others. After accepting the diagnosis, rehabilitative therapy is needed to retrain the body and mind. There are many ways to train one's body and mind, including medications, if needed. The process of rehabilitation, however, is long and arduous because the hurt psyche (mind) needs time to heal.

This book, which documents this painful process—a process still underway—will be very helpful to many patients who are suffering from the same disease but feel reluctant to discuss it.

Jeon Beomseok
Professor of Neurology at Seoul National University Hospital,
Chairman of the Local Organizing Committee of the
2025 World Congress of Neurology

In life, things happen unexpectedly. What would you do if one day a painful illness hit you all of a sudden? This book was written by sociologist and professor Shim Young-hee, who suffered from a rare disease called "functional movement disorder". This book, which includes her husband's contributions, chronicles her struggle with the disorder. In general, sociologists are not personally involved in the material they produce. However, in the pages that follow, the pain of the body and mind experienced by the author is described in a striking and detailed way. More importantly, it is a record of her healing process, progressing a bit at a time in the midst of pain. The patient's will to fight the disease, the devoted support of her family, including her son, daughter, daughter-in-law, grandson, and granddaughter, and the assistance of hospital doctors, physical therapists and caregivers, all played a major role during the process.

But the most important force in her recovery was the devoted care of her husband, sociologist and professor Han Sang-jin. Prof. Han completely altered his life posture while observing his wife's illness as an intimate witness, setting his own life aside to prioritize his wife's health. Spending nearly every day with his ailing wife, Prof. Han documented the couple's journey as he cared for her and supported her. (He dedicatedly washed her feet each evening with warm water, for example.) Their two children, witnessing their father's extreme dedication and sincerity, themselves joined in the caregiving process. Even Shim's physicians and therapists have noted her husband's meticulous medical documentation and caring attitude.

Written by a married couple who are both sociologists, the book makes you think, "How would I deal with such a disease if it struck me out of the blue?" After reading the book, however, the message that remained for me was that the ultimate power to defeat disease comes from 'love'.

Cheong Soo-bok
sociologist / writer, author of
Paris Diary: Hermitage and Transformation

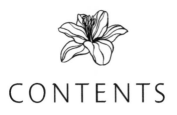

CONTENTS

. . .

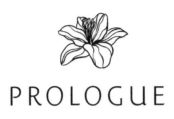

PROLOGUE

. . .

One Day, My Body Began to Scream

It was one day in 2017. I was having tea with my son's family after dinner.

"Mom, your head is shaking."

"Who, me? Is it? I don't think so."

Until I heard those words, I wasn't aware of any symptoms.

"Yeah, you're trembling . . ."

"It's nothing. It doesn't matter."

I was a little concerned, of course, but that's what I said anyway, lest the kids worry. If my eyelids were trembling, it would stop after a while. In my own way, I've always been confident when it comes to my health. I didn't take the matter seriously because up to that point I hadn't experienced any problems or impediments to my work.

A similar thing happened in 2018 when I was attending Mass at a Catholic church. My husband, standing next to me, whispered as he gently supported my back with his hand.

"Can't you just stand there without swaying?"

A Mass involves a lot of standing and sitting. My husband pointed out that while standing I kept moving my body forward and backward.

"Your body never stays still."

At this point, I began to feel a little worried.

When spring came, I told the attending physician at the hospital about these symptoms and he gave me a referral to the Department of Intractable Diseases. The doctor there examined me and listened to my health history, and without telling me what kind of disease it was, said that there was no need to take medication for the symptoms. I took that to mean it was no big deal, so I left it there.

It was early December, near the end of 2018. A couple, dear friends of ours for many years, came to visit and we were having tea together at a cafe near our house. We were sitting outside the cafe and it was a little chilly. Even though I didn't let on to the others, I was trembling so badly that my teeth started to rattle. It was nippy out, yes, but I was unaware at the time that the shivering might be caused by an illness. My body was definitely sending me a signal, but because of my 'old habit' of thinking that one's physical condition can be managed by one's own will power, I disregarded it.

We hadn't spoken in person in such a long time, we decided to catch up by strolling along the neighboring Picheondeuk Trail.

We talked and swapped memories well into the evening. It was late before we knew it, so I invited them to supper at my home. Despite the fact it was a very pleasant get-together and my spirits were high, my body felt cold and trembled as though I were suffering from a body ache.

At the end of June 2019, after receiving a diagnosis and a doctor's prescription, I went to the hair salon to get a perm. As the hairdresser started cutting my hair, I told her that my head might shake and make it challenging for her. She then said she'd noticed the shaking before, but hadn't brought it up. This proved that the symptoms existed before I became aware of them.

I began to worry about my health. Numerous things came into question, like the fact that I sleep on my left side most of the time. Was it connected to my symptoms? I started lying on my left side because sleeping that way promotes digestion and eases pressure on the stomach, which is located on the left side of the abdomen. Anyway, the claim seemed credible to me.

I eventually developed the habit of needing to sleep on my left side. Then one day, I realized I was losing strength in my left arm. Then it started feeling numb, my left shoulder hurt, and my left hand felt colder than my right hand. When I slept, I started to experience pressure on my left side. I questioned whether my nervous system was the cause of the problem.

When I was young, I often suffered from diarrhea, and even in college I always complained of stomach pains and headaches. But these were minor ailments. In fact, indigestion was a frequent cause of my headaches.

When I was studying in the U.S., I played tennis and exercised a lot, so I maintained a rather good level of health. Even after I became a professor, I walked back and forth to lunch on weekdays when I was on campus. At home on weekends, I didn't walk after meals and was apt to suffer from indigestion. I usually took a digestive tonic called *Hwalmyeongsu* that I purchased by the box. Anyway, since I was a kid, I had trouble with digestion and falling asleep. My health may have suffered as a result.

By the spring of 2019, the tremor was clearly noticeable. But I still didn't take it seriously. I believed it was just a case of the shakes and that it would pass quickly. After all, I'd already undergone a health checkup earlier that year, and had also received a diagnosis from a neurologist who assured me it was just a hand tremor.

At that time, I reported feeling a sudden loss of strength in my left arm, which got better, although a slight numbness persisted, and my hands felt cold. For that reason, a brain MRA was requested as an additional test. The doctor said that there was a bud-like cluster of blood vessels in my brain, but it was very tiny and posed no problem. The overall assessment was that the head tremor wasn't a huge matter and there was no need to be concerned.

But the tremor grew worse over time. My neck and back muscles violently contracted and knotted up. I was trembling so badly that it made me perspire and moving became difficult. I was admitted to the hospital again and underwent a thorough examination. My neck and back muscles were involuntarily contracting with violent spasms, and I wanted to know how to stop it. The biggest problem wasn't the insomnia; but if I lost sleep, my condition would worsen the next day, and the symptoms grew more severe over time.

Looking back, part of the problem was caused by the fact that I was overworked in the spring of 2019. I typically went to bed at two or three in the morning that semester. I couldn't sleep, even if I didn't drink coffee, if the slightest thing was bothering me. From February to May especially, my workload increased dramatically, and I got even less sleep than usual.

At the time, I was getting ready to publish a Korean translation of *La dynastie rouge* by the French historian Pascal Dayez-Burgeon. I proofread it five times by myself, in an effort to make a better book. If sleep wouldn't come, I'd work through the night; or I'd go to bed and wake up at the crack of dawn to continue working. The fifth and last revision was enough to make me sick. I'm fairly accustomed to reading on a daily basis, but this was the first time in my life that I experienced such a reaction. I worked very hard on the translation, but when the author came to Seoul in October, I was physically unable to attend any of the events, including the presentations the author gave.

Also, there was a succession of academic events taking place that spring. Following my presentation at an East Asian Sociological Association meeting in Japan, I met Japanese academics to discuss the new worldwide research network we'd launched. Immediately after that, I assisted in organizing an academic gathering for which a British sociologist had been invited. This event proved to be very demanding because we had to accompany him to several universities and locations. Early in May, my husband

and I had to host Chinese professors for a number of academic events and even give presentations in English.

By March, the body tremor had become much worse, and I experienced muscle contractions, making my neck and back uncomfortably stiff. The tremor was so violent that anyone holding my hand would feel it pulsate in their own body. Additionally, I would frequently get fevers because of the chaotic physical tos and fros. Even though summer was a long way off, I felt so hot that I couldn't survive without air conditioning. I sweated so much that the back of my head and neck were often dripping wet. Also, when I was lying down immobile for extended periods of time, I experienced constipation and had major difficulties using the restroom.

In addition, I had to make a presentation at the Joongmin Forum in May. The day of the presentation, my body was trembling, worsened by the fact that I hadn't gotten any sleep the night before. I could hardly function with all the throbbing and the stiffness. It made eating, using the computer, or composing an instant message on my cell phone all but impossible, let alone a public speech. My left shoulder hurt like it had never hurt before, and I was drenched in perspiration.

I couldn't go to my office anymore because I was physically exhausted. I was able to carry on with my daily activities up until April, but by mid-May, it was out of the question.

PART 1

. . .

Why Is This Happening to Me?

CHAPTER 1

. . .

"This Is Functional Movement Disorder Syndrome."

The Obscure Disease Called 'a Syndrome'

"Exactly what kind of disease is it? Does it have a name?"

Does Anyone Know About This Illness?

I SANK LIKE A CLUMP OF gray ash. On May 15, 2019, after exhausting all of my energy making a presentation for the "fiery" Joongmin Forum that year, my daily existence came to an end. Instead, angry muscles wrangled and clambered under my skin.

"It's not some serious disease, I hope?"

"Don't worry. You'll get an answer when you go to the hospital."

"What if it's Parkinson's, or . . . ?"

The names of all the diseases I knew began to flash through my head, and with each name, the fragmentary information I'd learned about each one heightened my fear, which was fast building up like a snowball. My terror was approaching the point of panic.

I knew I needed to visit a hospital, but I was unsure about which facility or type of physician to choose. When I did an online search of my symptoms, I couldn't figure out whether it was Parkinson's disease or simple tremors.

I personally or indirectly questioned a number of doctors about it. Several mentioned the medication Synthyroid, which I'd been taking since my 20s for hypothyroidism. They speculated that it might be a side effect of taking the medication in excess. So, from May 17, I cut my thyroid medication dosage in half.

The next day, I tried getting a massage from a masseur, a sight-impaired gentleman, in hopes that loosening up my tight muscles would increase the blood flow in my body. I also noticed that a few days of riding a stationary bike at the gym reduced the tremors. I made a note to myself that regular exercise might also help.

Later, by chance, I learned about the renowned Parkinson's specialist, Professor Jeon Beomseok. I learned about Prof. Jeon from a married couple living in the United Arab Emirates who were my former students and whose wedding I'd officiated. The wife was working at Sheikh Khalifa Hospital, which was commissioned to run by Seoul National University Hospital.

Every time the couple came back to Seoul, they would drop by to say hello and we'd have dinner together. When they came to visit in mid-March, I decided to ask them about my symptoms during our chitchat. I reasoned that since the wife is a neurosurgeon, she might know something about it. Shortly after arriving back in the UAE, she wrote me a 'Kakao Talk' message, outlining her research on the tremor and mentioning Prof. Jeon at Seoul National University Hospital. She said nothing about Parkinson's disease, probably wanting to keep things pleasant.

I looked up Prof. Jeon online and discovered that he was a true survivor and champion. He had severely damaged his spinal cord during a mountain climbing fall, but he was able to walk again thanks to his solid determination and the work he put into his rehabilitation activities. He ultimately rose to prominence as a leading authority on Parkinson's disease. I needed to see this person for therapy, I thought.

The appointment was set for 11:30 am on May 20. There were a number of people waiting to see the neurologist when I arrived at the hospital. Appointments were behind schedule. My body grew increasingly uncomfortable, and I tried to ease the boredom by sitting, standing, and walking up and down the hallway. It turned out that my 11:30 appointment was the last schedule for him. I had to wait an additional hour and a half before I could see the doctor.

A person who seemed to be a resident confirmed my identity and immediately told me to try walking.

"Raise your hands."

"Now, twist your wrists like you're waving your hands."

"Make two fists, then spread out your fingers."

I did my best and successfully performed the movements he requested. Then the doctor, who had been watching, instructed me to visit the family medicine department since I didn't require a specialist's care. It was just a hand tremor.

"Huh? Is that all?" The disappointing diagnosis left me stunned, not relieved. I'd patiently awaited the scheduled appointment day. How much time had I spent getting ready to come to the hospital that morning, and even more after I arrived! After waiting for more than an hour and a half, I saw the doctor for no more than two or three minutes before being sent to see someone else. I stood there stock-still, exhausted and dejected, unsure of what to do.

It was time to leave the doctor's office. My husband, who was standing next to me, then explained that the muscles in my neck and back had been convulsing and knotting up. The doctor then instructed me to remove my outerwear and sit back down. As I was sitting there in my undershirt, Prof. Jeon asked the resident to video the muscle movements on my neck and back for the hospital's future use.

The doctor took a few moments to consider my condition and conceded that if things were as bad as all that, I'd need to be hospitalized and put through testing. With that, he sent an email to a professor he knew at Hallym University Sacred Heart Hospital in Pyeongchon, requesting a brain wave scan and an electromyogram. We applied to Seoul National University Hospital, requesting admittance as soon as a room became available.

The following day, I went directly to Hallym University Sacred Heart Hospital without scheduling an appointment, rather than waiting for admission at Seoul National University Hospital, which would take more than a week. The distance to the hospital was considerable. After a brief wait, I was given outpatient treatment and a test date was scheduled for three days later. On the test day, I returned and had the brain wave scan, and the professor came in person to do the electromyogram, which required puncturing my skin with a needle-like device. Because my muscle spasm was so active—exceeding once every three seconds—the measurement couldn't be taken. Nothing more could be done, so I returned home.

The Illness I Wish I Didn't Know About

T HE DATE WAS MAY 26. The whole family rallied together at the news of my scheduled hospitalization. Thankfully, I was notified that a room had become available at Seoul National University Hospital. I went through the admissions process and entered the room at 2:00 pm. I didn't give much consideration to the situation at first, but when I donned the patient gown, everyone commented that I really looked the part of a patient. The family went home and later, my daughter came to stay with me during the night.

My body shook incessantly, and even though the room wasn't warm, I sweat through my gown. At 5:00 pm, a nurse tried to read my blood pressure, but my spasms were too intense. I tried to hold my arm steady but couldn't. It was challenging for both of us, and after several failed attempts, the nurse gave up and left, saying she'd try again later.

In addition, plasma was drawn from my arm for a blood test, and a contrast medium was injected for the spine MRI. At 9:00 pm, I went for the MRI. The test looks for minute lesions and abnormalities, but my body kept thrashing about and the screening failed. At 11:00 pm, the nurse came back to check my blood pressure. It was nighttime and the spasms seemed to have calmed down a bit, so she finally managed to get the reading. Even the test preparation procedures proved to be exceedingly challenging.

On May 27, after eating porridge in the morning, I had to begin fasting. I wasn't allowed to consume any food or liquids. After the failed effort at getting the MRI the day before, I had to fast once again in order to get the sedative needed to manage the tremors. At 8:00 am, the attending physician came and conducted a physical examination. The blood pressure reading was 139/80. My son purchased cup noodles for us to share, but I couldn't eat.

At 1:40 pm, consent forms for a sedation and colonoscopy were presented and signed. During my medical checkup in January, several polyps had been detected. Several of them were removed at that time, and the other ones were scheduled for surgery on this visit. At 9:40 pm, the attending physician announced that the colonoscopy scheduled for the next day would be postponed by 24 hours. He said that for the endoscopy, I had to receive sedative injections that would interfere with the brain wave scan. As a result, the length of my hospitalization and fasting period were extended by one day. At 11:15 pm, I was sedated and the MRI was performed successfully.

On May 28, I was put on an IV drip from 4:00 am to 6:30 am. At 12:45 pm, I was instructed to go to the fourth floor in a short-sleeved gown and knee-length shorts. My son, who was visiting, went with me. While waiting, Prof. Jeon and the residents decided to videotape the exam. They had me walk, sit in a chair, and pretend to eat, and I made an effort to carry out each motion. I could lift my arm and mimic holding a spoon while pretending to eat, but when I tried to eat actual food, I couldn't manage. What was happening . . . !

At 1:00 pm, they performed the brain scan—similar to what they did at the Pyeongchon hospital but with considerably greater care. Due to the exam, I missed Prof. Jeon's 2 o'clock round. At 3:10, another doctor, who appeared to work under Prof. Jeon, arrived and left after a few minutes, and at 5 o'clock I drank my first dose of coolprep acid as a bowel wash in preparation for the colonoscopy.

I had only eaten porridge that day, twice in the morning and again in the afternoon. Maybe that's why I was weak and I needed an IV. At 10:00 pm, I took another dose of coolprep acid. From midnight, I had to fast again—no food or liquids.

On May 29, a nurse came at 5:00 am, informed me that the endocrine examination had revealed no abnormalities, and gave me the same medications as before, including thyroid medication, high blood pressure medication, blood clotting medication, and Dicamax. A doctor arrived at 9:00 am and reported that the brain scan and spinal MRI were good, and that the thyroid test was normal. At 4:20 pm, I moved to another room to receive a colonoscopy under sedation.

Finally, at 6:00 pm, Prof. Jeon came and gave a thorough explanation of the test results. It appeared that he went in more depth since my husband was in the room. When all the test findings were taken into account, he said, there was no structural issue, but there was a functional issue that was likely brought on by 'stress'. Knowing that I'm a professor, he added, "You've been doing research all your life. It's certainly not your research putting you through this kind of stress." He was as baffled as I was, as to why I'd developed the symptoms so suddenly. Upon hearing this, my husband asked,

"Exactly what kind of disease is it? Does it have a name?"

"You can say it's a psychogenic illness. The term used recently is Functional Movement Disorder."

"And after the stress you referred to goes away, she'll get better . . . ?"

"Right now, it's difficult to say. But she'll have to relearn every aspect of daily living, including breathing, walking, sitting, and eating."

Prof. Jeon said that the condition was uncommon, so there were few scholarly studies and no known treatments. He recommended physical therapy as the best course of action for managing the symptoms. He said that as far as he knew, Professor Park Jung E of Dongguk University's Ilsan Hospital was the only doctor who'd ever treated it. Prof. Jeon then said that he'd write to Prof. Park and request a referral. He then asked me to schedule a follow-up appointment with him in three months and report on my progress at that time.

At 10:30 pm, a nurse arrived to get me ready for my discharge. She gave me the referral, confirmed my appointment, and informed me that I'd be discharged the following day after eating and getting checked for rectal bleeding. Around 11:00 pm my IV was removed. They offered to let me stay on the IV longer, but I declined. I don't like getting stuck with needles and didn't want to prolong my stay. Knowing the disease's name made it even more frustrating. I'd just undergone a grueling battery of tests with no conclusive result, and now I had to go to another hospital for more care. A big hassle.

Fortunately, there was no blood in my stool, and so on May 30, I was finally discharged from the hospital. At 10:45 am, the nurse brought me some endocrine medication. At noon I had a meal with rice and took a short stroll down the corridor and back with my daughter. I was discharged at 1:30 pm. My daughter had come and stayed every night during my hospitalization. What a wonderful daughter!

The Correlation between Muscle Tremors and the Mind

"I came to the conclusion after reading these papers that FMD, a condition only lately given a name, is difficult to explain to patients."

Stress Is the King of All Diseases

ANOTHER DISAPPOINTINGLY BRIEF DIAGNOSIS. I'd undergone testing and hospitalization and was looking forward to a definitive answer that would give me some hope for the future. Instead, I received a desultory discharge. My frustration and anxiety soared to an even higher level than before hospitalization. What on earth was this 'Functional Movement Disorder'? It was something totally foreign to me.

I quickly looked through a number of web portals but to no avail. I searched a bit more on Google and discovered a few papers. I skipped over the medical ones that were too complicated for me to understand, and picked out a few that might help me learn more about Functional Movement Disorder.

That's when I came across a paper published in 2014 titled "From Psychogenic Movement Disorder to Functional Movement Disorder: It's Time to Change the Name".[1]

---

[1] "From Psychogenic Movement Disorder to Functional Movement Disorder: It's Time to Change the Name", Mark J. Edwards PhD, Jon Stone PhD, Anthony E. Lang MD, *Movement Disorders* 29(7), June 2014, pp.849–852.

The word 'psychogenic' was cited in the research as the most frequently used term to describe aberrant motor signs of the body. The authors claimed that the label "psycho-genic", which implies that the symptom is "in the mind", already poses a challenge to assigning a cause to the disease.

Above all, they said, because the syndrome hasn't been adequately pinpointed, medical professionals should avoid using terms based on ill-defined causative theories, and instead refer to patients as having a 'functional disorder'.

Even in this article, I had trouble finding the answers I was looking for. The muscles of my body weren't throbbing as a result of my conscious volition or thought, so I could understand the argument that the term 'psychogenic' wasn't applicable. Nonetheless, it was difficult to see why the definition of the abnormal movement symptoms had to be widened using the word 'functional'. To a patient who was interested in learning the source of her illness, it appeared evasive.

Another paper I read was "How Do I Explain the Diagnosis of Functional Movement Disorder to a Patient?" published in 2019.[2] According to this article, Functional Movement Disorder or FMD is a well-recognized cause of severe pain and disability, and a common phenomenon in neurological practice. Many doctors, however, have had trouble explaining the diagnosis to their patients. The article also made note of the fact that because it can be difficult to make a precise diagnosis, a propensity exists to

---

[2] "How Do I Explain the Diagnosis of Functional Movement Disorder to a Patient?", Jon Stone FRCP PhD, Ingrid Hoeritzauer MB BCh MRCP, *Movement Disorders* 6(5), June 2019, p.419.

emphasize psychological factors rather than assisting patients in understanding the nature and mechanism of the disorder itself.

I had the impression that each doctor, as they made their individual assessment, was considering the same issues as I was. Even medical professionals appeared to struggle to identify symptoms that have no known cause. Although the disease was difficult to comprehend, it seemed that doctors were saying that in order to solve the diagnostic conundrum, one should not only concentrate on psychological causes, but also make sure that patients are aware of the cyclical mechanism associated with the treatments for the disorder. These treatments, they claimed, stimulate the brain, which causes the body to return to normal. The mind is likewise affected, which in turn improves the treatment prognosis.

I became increasingly perplexed. I came to the conclusion after reading these papers that FMD, a condition only lately given a name, is difficult to explain to patients. The fact that after extensive testing, the doctor was unable to identify the illness with any degree of scientific certainty, referring to it as a psychogenic disease and often using the word "stress" in his explanations, gave me the main gist. In the end, stress is the 'alpha and omega' of every illness!

By the time I found myself in the hospital, the situation set to unfold seemed strangely out of the ordinary. It became obvious that things were only going to get worse. The Saint-Émilion conference, scheduled for the end of June, was drawing near. Participants from all over the world would present and discuss papers on the subject of 'alternative social theory' during the conference, which would take the form of a workshop. My husband

and I were invited to the conference and had already booked our plane tickets.

Even better, for the duration of our stay, the host gave us free use of a property in a small Bordeaux-region community known for its wineries. I'd never been to Bordeaux, and as it was close to Saint-Jean-Pied-de-Port, the starting point of the Santiago pilgrimage, I'd made the decision, before my illness got bad, to take the opportunity to walk the pilgrimage route.

My Life Is Destroyed and My Dreams Vanish

I HAD A BURNING DESIRE TO make the Santiago pilgrimage for a long time. I found, read, and saw television shows and documentaries about the pilgrimage route. I'd also enquired about it to a friend from my all-girls high school who had undergone cancer surgery and had gone there twice. I looked up the best route from Bordeaux to Saint-Jean-Pied-de-Port on a map. I could walk for a day or two, and give up if it proved too difficult. Just starting the pilgrimage would fulfill a big dream of mine.

Because Bordeaux, where we would be staying, is in the southwest of France, and Marseille is in the southeast, we'd be able to cut through not only Aix-en-Provence, where we visit every year, but also Toulouse and Montpellier, places where we'd never been. I had high hopes.

Why did I have such a strong desire to walk the Camino de Santiago? In hindsight, I believe it was because I'd lived my life with my eyes fixed forward and because I wanted to have time to reflect on myself. What did I dream of? What had I in mind to do?

I was once asked why I applied to the English department by a university admissions reviewer. I answered with confidence that I wished to travel the world as a journalist, learn five languages, and write a book based on my experiences. Yet, I'm a sociologist. That's not bad, and you could say that I've achieved my own measure of success. I made a small contribution to raising awareness of sexual violence as a societal issue in Korea through my early studies on the subject.

What did I want now, though, in the midst of illness? I wanted to think back on my past, carefully evaluating everything I'd missed out on. I genuinely wondered what I'd learn if I put everything aside and made a physically taxing trek.

Despite my best efforts, my functional movement disorder blocked any route to the Camino de Santiago. I informed our hosts that my body was acting strangely. I'd been admitted to the hospital for tests, and I couldn't attend in my present condition. My husband asked if he should also skip the event since I couldn't go. I strongly advised him to make the trip because there were no other Koreans among the participants. My husband left on schedule for France while my daughter agreed to look after me at home.

Let's Do Everything We Can

"How is it now? Does it feel any better now?"
"I don't know. I wish you'd do it a little harder."

Can I Get Better with Medication Alone?

AFTER BEING RELEASED FROM THE hospital, I went to see Prof. Park Jung E at Dongguk University Hospital on June 3, at the recommendation of Prof. Jeon. She was the sole provider of FMD physiotherapy. It was a challenge just to get to Ilsan, which is somewhat remote from my home in Seoul.

"There is no prescribed physical therapy for functional movement disorder."

"Then what should I do?"

On the first visit, my hopes that Prof. Park would be able to relieve the tremors in my neck and back, both hard as a block of stone, vanished like a bubble.

After examining the referral paperwork and assessing my health, the doctor informed me that the 'physical therapy' I would receive was strictly for research purposes and not for commercial use. She said that the disease is psychogenic and prescribed 0.25 mg doses of Alpram, a stabilizer and muscle relaxant, to be taken in the morning, at lunch, and at dinner. Regarding the course of scheduled office visits, she said initially it would be once every two weeks, then once a month, and finally once every two months.

"Anyway, as things stand now, there's nothing you can do other than take medication to help relieve the symptoms."

"When can I expect improvement?"

Prof. Park offered some hope, saying that I might see improvement in three to six months. She went on to say that yoga and extensive meditation would be beneficial. The idea that I had to take 'psychiatric medications' and had no choice but to hope for improvement through yoga and meditating instead of physical therapy, was demoralizing.

Between the diagnosis and the first treatment, I experienced no major problems with sitting or moving around. When my two students came to visit on June 8, I shook a little but otherwise had no issues as we enjoyed lunch and tea outside. My older brother and his wife stopped by to see us the following day, and everything was still okay. That evening we went to offer our condolences to the family members of Lee Hee-ho, wife of the late President Kim Dae-jung, who had passed away.

I saw the movie *Parasite* a few days later with my daughter-in-law, and even then, moving around wasn't too difficult. I thought that as time went on, my condition would get better a little at a time.

Then, on June 15, the newly appointed president of the Girls' High School Professionals' Association, for which I had previously served as the founding president, called me. She invited me to an upcoming meeting at her Pyeongchang-dong home. I politely declined her invitation, with a detailed explanation of my circumstances. She suggested that I could just show up for a little while and leave early, but she really wanted me to come.

I couldn't say no to her because she'd previously supported me greatly when I was president, both materially and spiritually.

About 30 members were present at the gathering. I was so pleased to see everybody after such a long time, I couldn't just show up and leave immediately. Refusing the luncheon that had been painstakingly prepared and served under a shade canopy set up in the beautiful garden, wasn't an easy task. Deciding that I could wait a bit longer before leaving, I took a fork from the table with my left hand and started eating.

We took a group photo at the top of a large rocky hill in the garden after lunch before going for a walk. This was immediately followed by a performance by two vocalists accompanied by piano. It was even harder for me to leave during a performance, so I waited there what was probably two hours. I could feel myself trembling a little at that point, but nothing really bad.

By the end of June, the situation changed dramatically. June 27 was the day our female professors' group decided to have a get-together for lunch, and despite experiencing some minor shaking, I attended. Everyone was worried because I held my fork awkwardly in my left hand as I ate, since I normally use my right hand when using chopsticks. In fact, I took great care to hide the tremors whenever I moved my arm or hand. I didn't want to make everyone uneasy.

I struggled to sit still as my body and mind grew more and more tense, so I got up to leave before everyone else. When I stopped by the bathroom on my way out, my face in the mirror looked pale and bloodless. It took me aback.

Despite taking the medication as directed, things continued to worsen. It was so difficult and so painful while my husband was away in France that, on Saturday, June 29, ahead of my scheduled appointment, I hastily made an appointment for myself and went to the hospital with my daughter. However, there was no solution other than changing my Alpram dosage.

On June 30, my daughter suggested that we see a movie—something we hadn't done in a while—so we went to check out the live-action film version of *Aladdin*. My body had been feeling so listless, I went along, just for a change in atmosphere. I was able to sit still at first, but soon my entire body began pulsating erratically. Even though the air conditioner in the theater was on and it was chilly inside, I felt like I was in a sauna, I was perspiring so heavily. It wasn't easy to leave in the middle of the film, so I waited out the two hours, which felt like ten, struggling and unsure of what to do.

Meditation, Yoga, Massages, and Acupressure

WHEN I STARTED TO GET seriously and visibly ill, my family started looking for anything and everything that could help me.

Prof. Park had recommended meditation, so my son came and meditated with me. It would benefit him as well, he said. He made a point of stopping by the apartment every day after lunch. We probably did 'Healing Meditation' 20 times together.

I could lie still initially and follow along because the meditations lasted only about 20 minutes, but with each passing day, they grew longer. As my condition worsened, I was having spasms so badly that I couldn't lie still. I ultimately gave up on meditation.

Prof. Park also recommended yoga, so I visited a "yoga academy" on June 12 and discussed my condition with the instructors there. I applied for a high-end yoga class that was taught by the director. I chose to go on Tuesdays and Thursdays twice a week, but it was difficult to do it alone, so I decided to go once a week on my own and once a week with my daughter.

I took my first class on June 18 and my second one on June 20. We began with exercises that involved stretching the upper and lower body in opposite directions, after which we studied poses like the cat pose, snake pose, dog pose, and tree pose. I kept with it and the yoga instructor encouraged me to keep advancing, saying that my body was supple and that I was following along well.

However, after being brought by ambulance to the emergency room for constipation on July 4, it became harder to do the yoga. I attended a yoga session on July 9 and left exhausted, and on July 11, my neck stiffened and my general health visibly declined.

On July 16, I couldn't even eat dinner because I was so worn-out from my yoga lesson.

At first, I could walk to class, but later I was unable to walk far and had to go back and forth by car. It became more and more difficult for me to make it to the yoga studio, and when I did make it, I'd come home so tired that I found myself lying sprawled out on the floor and unable to eat dinner. When I completed nine of the twelve classes I'd planned to take, I made the decision to stop and promised to come back when I felt better.

As time went on, my back muscles began to twitch and pulsate uncontrollably, then gradually started to toughen and harden as a result of the constant uncontrolled muscle activity. The longer this carried on, the more unsettled my thinking became. I was unable to touch the affected muscles myself, but my family members said that when they applied significant pressure on my back, the muscles wouldn't yield in the slightest.

Ultimately, the doctor advised acupressure or massages to help reduce my back pain, and so on June 4 I began receiving acupressure at a facility that my son's friend had recommended. My son said that receiving acupressure there had relieved his excruciating leg pain. I'd also used acupressure in the past for back pain and leg pain. I started receiving acupressure treatments, first daily and then three times each week, to see if they would help.

The acupressure specialist was in Mapo, roughly 40 minutes away from my apartment building. I needed a car. After totaling his previous vehicle in 2018 in a collision caused by a sudden acceleration, my husband bought a new one and hired a driver named Mr. Kim to help drive it.

My brother-in-law later informed me of my husband's decision. My husband promised he'd do anything to make sure I recover when I first started feeling ill. That must have been why he purchased a new car and hired a driver. It shocked me to learn this about my ever-frugal husband. I simply couldn't picture him doing it. Previously, my nephew had driven me around, but once we purchased the new car, Mr. Kim helped me. The passenger seat in the new car didn't recline all the way back, but we quickly had it fixed so that it could.

I rode in the car almost flat on my back, with the passenger seat reclined all the way down. The driver hung several straps from the hook above the car window for me to hold on to; otherwise, I wouldn't be able to lie still. As we traveled, I alternately grabbed the front and back straps with my right hand. The sky was all I could see, yet I was unconcerned with either it or myself as I watched it pass swiftly by.

Most of the time, we took the Mapo Bridge over the Han River from the Olympic Expressway, but we sometimes crossed the Dongjak Bridge and took the Gangbyeon North Road, which felt like a longer route. It was challenging to get out of the car, ride the elevator to the second floor, get treated, then return to the first floor and take the several steps down from the entranceway.

It saddened Mr. Kim, the driver, to see my condition getting worse day by day.

"Tell me if you feel pain."

During the entire session, the acupressure therapist asked me how my body was reacting.

"It's okay. I still don't feel anything."

It might have been 10 out of 10, for all I knew. All I discerned was discomfort. When one side of my back became a wee more relaxed, the other side would grow stiff. I asked for permission to lie on my side during treatment because I found the prone position to be very painful. Yet, it still wasn't comfortable, even in that position.

"How is it now? Does it feel any better now?"

"I don't know. I wish you'd do it a little harder."

The therapist became drenched in perspiration as he worked, but I didn't experience any pain. I hardly felt anything at all. He tried putting my arms in different positions and pressing my shoulders in different ways, but confessed he had trouble locating the acupoints.

My shoulders and neck appeared to ease up a little when the therapist placed my arms behind my neck and performed a concentrated adjustment, tightening and loosening my shoulders with a "pop". Yet, while it was pleasant enough during the therapy, it grew worse again when I got home after the long, uncomfortable ride in the car. This happened numerous times.

My husband said that while the acupressure itself was alright, the prolonged car trip afterward wasn't. After some research, he scheduled an appointment with a blind masseur in Bukchang-dong, who was reputed to be quite skilled, to massage me at our home. The driver brought the masseur in the evening after regular business hours, and took him back when the massage was finished. We did it at the foot of our bed initially, but I later purchased a massage bed to give the masseur fuller and freer movement.

The masseur was motivated at first, but after failing three or four times, he gave up. He would work vigorously to release my tense muscles, but the severity of the muscle spasms just increased when he did. It was like a wall shifting around, he said, a kind of "balloon effect" of the muscles.

When he loosened one side, the other side would harden up; then when he loosened that area, the other area would twitch and get puffy. No matter how hard he tried to relieve my stiffness, it was impossible to relax all areas at once.

The masseur said that my case was a very unusual one and that I wasn't responding to his massages. If he were to massage his other clients with full vigor, they'd cry out in mortal anguish. I felt no pain at all, though, which was really surprising. That's how stiff my back muscles were. They appeared to resist, to harden, as a response to being rubbed.

The just-stimulated muscles would actually throb more violently than usual at night and grow heavy and rigid. The pain, stiffness, and strain made falling sleep very difficult. I'd toss and turn, get up, wander around, then lie down again and continue tossing and turning. At those times, the medications were of no use. Finally, I gave up on massage therapy.

CHAPTER 2

. . .

*Daily Life with Tremors, Stiffness,
and Paralysis*

A Physical System Out of Control

"My neck and back were throbbing so hard that I thought I'd go crazy, and my body felt heavy with an excruciating ache, as if I were being crushed by a rock."

Being Taken to the ER by Ambulance for Constipation

THUD! I WAS SO WORN out that I passed out on the bathroom floor. I got up on the morning of July 4 and went to the bathroom, but despite my best efforts, no stool came out. Constipation! As a child, I'd endured recurrent diarrhea, for which my mother frequently gave me a bitter decoction of motherwort, but I'd never suffered constipation. However, it was quite serious now, because I wasn't moving around much due to my condition.

For a while, I sat by myself, moving my body in various directions as I contemplated my options. I was shivering and perspiring, and I strained so much that my face was burning. My body was clammy with sweat. Perspiration dripped down my forehead. I tried to recall if I'd put this much effort giving birth. I tried once, took a rest, then tried again over a dozen times, but my bowels would not move. Frustrated, I was about to give up and get up from the toilet, but I had no energy to do so. For a time, my head swam. Just as I decided that calling out to my sleeping husband would be going too far, my body collapsed.

My husband woke up in surprise at the sound and came running.

"Hey, you should have called me. What's going on?"

My husband, understanding the predicament, tried to help me by getting a suppository, but it didn't help. While getting me to the bedroom, he insisted we go to the hospital. I couldn't even stand up without help, much less walk alone. My body was completely out of my control.

Some time passed. In the morning, my son, who lives in the same building, came up to see us. He called an ambulance after seeing my weakened state, pointing out that in my condition, traveling to the hospital by car would be impossible. Soon, the paramedics came. I'd barely put on my coat when I was lifted onto a stretcher and taken to the ambulance.

Since only one guardian could accompany me in the ambulance, my son went with me and my husband followed in his car. I closed my eyes because I was in such pain.

"Ma'am, open your eyes. Open your eyes, please."

The paramedic periodically checked on me en route to the hospital. He instructed me to keep my eyes open. He must have thought I'd passed out. St. Mary's Hospital was nearby, but it was only taking patients with life-threatening emergencies. I was brought instead to the emergency room at Chung-Ang University Hospital.

When I got there, the hospital staff first took abdominal X-rays. The doctor finally arrived and examined the results. He said that my intestines were too full and remarked in a regretful tone that I must have had quite an urge to evacuate my bowels. It's hard to put it into words how serious the situation was on that day. As the doctor treated me, he added that he'd never seen such acute constipation. It must have been hard for my husband to stand there and see so much that he didn't need to see. He said it was surprising that there could be so much feces in a human body. When I left the emergency room, I had no shoes on. I'd come by ambulance stretcher so I hadn't put any on. I eventually made it home in just my sock feet.

The problem began after I got home. I had to eat something before taking the medicine prescribed by the hospital. I had to sit down to eat but my body felt so weak, I couldn't control my motions. My body was like a jellyfish pulled from the water.

Even with my husband holding me in his arms and my daughter spooning rice gruel into my mouth, swallowing was no mean feat. I couldn't even get one spoonful down before passing out. After getting back on the chair, I still couldn't eat the gruel, so I ate a chunk of watermelon instead. The watermelon was cool to the tongue and easy to swallow.

Three spoonsful of rice and three chunks of melon were all I could manage to get down before I collapsed again, unable to eat any more. Then, at last, I took the medicine. I was in the worst state imaginable. Seeing this, my husband cautioned me that I needed to regain my energy and began urging me to keep walking.

Insomnia, the Terrible Sleep Disorder

To compound the problem, my insomnia got worse. Maybe all the sleep deprivation contributed to the disease. Staying up late was an old, bad habit of mine. Second, I hadn't been able to sleep much because I had so much work to complete between February and May of that year.

The problem was that I still had trouble falling asleep, even after taking the medication the hospital had prescribed. Even after taking Rivotril, the drug I took for sleeplessness, there were now more nights when I struggled to fall asleep. I wasn't sure if the worsening insomnia was a side effect of the medication or a reaction to it. I had no idea what was taking place inside my body.

I had to eat dinner, take a pill, and wait about an hour and a half before I could go to sleep. That was on days when I was in good condition. Very frequently, I had to take an additional pill when sleep wouldn't come.

I would frequently try to escape the awful body tremors, by taking medicine and going out like a light. It was stressful when I tried to sleep without the extra dose, and stressful when I took the extra dose but still had trouble dropping off.

When I went to bed, I made an effort to unwind as much as I could. It was, however, suffocating as the muscles in my neck began to jerk frantically, pulling my neck about as if to choke me. My back muscles repeatedly pounded and throbbed violently, lumping up like hard, frozen snowballs. My neck and back were throbbing so hard that I thought I'd go crazy, and my body felt heavy with an excruciating ache, as if I were being crushed by a rock. It was like a bully beating me up. I was being drawn into a swamp from which there was no way to escape.

While I tossed and turned in agony, my husband helped me in doing all the stretches I could. If those didn't work, he either got out of bed and went to his study, or stayed there until I fell asleep.

There was nothing else to do but break down and cry on nights when neither of those solutions worked. I cried like a baby before drifting off to sleep. My husband tried his best to calm me down by giving me hugs, wiping away my tears, and singing "The Lord's Prayer" with me during those moments, but there was basically nothing he could do.

I eventually ended up with my head at the foot of the bed, and my legs toward the pillows because the tossing and turning lasted no matter how much I changed my sleeping position. My daughter would come and wash my face with some Eau de toilette, apply lotion, and then help do arm rotations or rowing motions to relax my tense muscles before I settled down for the night.

My husband slept in the same direction as me. He could then assist me when I couldn't sleep, or when I got up in the middle of the night and had trouble falling back asleep, by helping me rotate my arm or do rowing motions. When I slept with my head at the foot of the bed, my husband would sometimes sit on a chair facing me and assist me with my arm exercises. Doing so let me spread out more than when I slept the regular way. It was very worrying, indeed regrettable, that my husband was also suffering, as he wouldn't fall asleep until he was certain I was.

Neck Tremors, Stiff Back Muscles, and Sweating

AS MY GENERAL STATE WORSENED, my husband decided to take a video of the muscle tremors on my neck and back. His diary reads as follows:

> "When my wife urinates in the bathroom, the motions of her body as she tears off the toilet paper or flushes the toilet are so unnaturally stiff, it's like watching a cartoon. The motions do not connect naturally and are like a series of separate disjointed actions. This is bizarre physical behavior. I wanted to be able to monitor how her condition was changing, so I captured her neck tremors on camcorder. The right side seems much worse than the left. Her neck feels tight and is inflexible. It is very difficult to manually relieve her neck pain."

I gave Prof. Park my husband's notes on July 16 during my visit to her office. The notes summed up the video and my daily physical condition, my medical history, the progression of my treatment and the medications I was prescribed, my urgent questions and needs as a patient, and the things the patient wanted to know:

> "First, about her physical tremors. She had no significant issues with sitting or walking prior to her first treatment on June 3, but she now frequently needs to lie down due to the acute spasms and stiffness in the back muscles that connect to her neck. These make sitting

difficult. But even when lying down, she is unable to lie still, and moves her arms and legs and turns her body from side to side, maybe in response to the functional movement disorder.

Eating, drinking, taking a shower, brushing her teeth, etc. have all become exceedingly tough tasks for her to perform with her hands. As a result, she has an extremely challenging daily life. It takes a lot of work for her to talk, and at times she finds doing so uncomfortable. More and more often, family members have to put food in my wife's mouth at mealtimes. She still struggles to swallow food and perspires a lot as she struggles. Her neck muscles quake when she drinks water, so drinking must be done quickly and with great effort. Despite the treatment, her illness seems to worsen rather than improve.

Second, the current state of her medical care and medication: Her prescribed medication was changed to be taken only once in the morning, but the symptoms have gotten worse at night, making her neck and lower body rigid and giving her sleep problems. She has used Alpram to get to sleep for the last three days. She does yoga twice a week for an hour with a qualified instructor in Bangbae-dong. She was flexible and seemed to do very well when she and the director performed yoga on a one-to-one basis. The instructor said as much. Yet after an hour of yoga, she gets very tired and her neck muscles are activated, making it impossible for her to eat dinner and forcing her to lie down.

*Questions: Would Botox injections help calm the
aberrant muscle movements? Should she continue using
Alpram and other muscle relaxants? Would you deem the
given medication to be effective? Yoga was recommended,
but there are significant negative side effects. Should she
continue? Could it possibly make matters worse?"*

After watching the video, Prof. Park suggested a Huntington
genetic test, just in case, possibly because she found it concerning.
According to her, the test is performed when 'chorea' is suspected,
a disorder in which a patient's body jerks uncontrollably as though
dancing. I questioned her about some treatment-related details
I'd discovered since my previous visit. A Botox injection was
given to a friend of mine every few months to cure her twitching
eyelids. I pondered whether getting Botox would be beneficial
because I was going through a particularly terrible time in my
daily life. Prof. Park indicated that while in many cases Botox
would be helpful, it wouldn't in my case because the extent of my
muscle tremors was so broad. She concluded that taking such a
step would be unwise.

That day my prescriptions increased from two to three. I was
to continue taking the antidepressant Lexapro and the muscle
relaxant Alpram, and add an anticonvulsant called Rivotril. All
three medications were to be taken starting that day. She advised
me to take Alpram in the evening, Rivotril when I couldn't sleep
at night, and Lexapro and Rivotril in the morning. After two
months, she said, I should be able to see a difference.

I was too worn out to eat dinner when I got home from the appointment. For several days, my stiff neck made it difficult to sit for very long, and it was equally hard to stand and walk. I frequently had to lie down because of the terrible cramping and stiffness in the back muscles leading up to my neck. This made it impossible to sit comfortably. But even in a lying position, there were tremors in my hands and feet and my body swayed from side to side, possibly due to the FMD.

I hoped to get some actual "therapy" after a few days of this. On July 23, I went to see a professor at Gangnam St. Mary's Hospital's Department of Rehabilitation Medicine. The day of my first visit, I had to spend a lot of time getting all the medical records from Seoul National University Hospital transferred, as well as conducting the patient interview, only to learn that there was no rehabilitation program there for patients like me.

Yet, because I was already there, I inquired about the physical therapy options. I was informed that they use electricity, however, which wouldn't be very helpful. According to Mr. Kim, our driver, who later did some research, the neurologists at St. Mary's and at other hospitals use electricity in the majority of their treatments. It was only the orthopedic doctors who used physical therapy, in their one-on-one manual therapy rehabilitation program.

The Fear of Paralysis Becomes a Reality

". . . I might actually experience the terrifying state of being unable to move my body as I want. No, it was already happening."

My Arms, Fingers, Neck, Mouth and Tongue Harden

THE TREMORS AND THE STIFFNESS in my neck and back muscles began to affect other parts of my body as well. From the neck upwards, all functioning deteriorated, and below the neck, normal movement was hindered in my extremities—shoulders, back, arms, and even fingers. My upper body motor functions and other related functions were overall impaired.

The stiffness and tremors weren't the only issue. My fingers began to numb and lose their range of motion, and my right arm began to feel heavy like a barbell and stiffen like a board.

Anxiety and fear engulfed me more and more. Everything that required me to use my hands, arms, or neck, including eating, drinking water, taking a shower, and brushing my teeth, became all but impossible at this point. I worried that I might actually experience the terrifying state of being unable to move my body as I want. No, it was already happening.

It eventually got to the point where I couldn't even raise a spoon, so I had to let others feed me. Since I was unable to sit on a chair, I stood leaning on a walker in front of a folding tray placed on top of the dining table. After I opened my mouth and said "ah", my daughter would put food in my mouth. Despite my best efforts to steady myself and keep my mouth open, very little food actually made it down my throat.

Because of the tremors, I found it difficult to keep my mouth open and chew well enough to swallow the food. And the whole time, the sweat just poured and poured. Sometimes, soaked in perspiration from exercising the sheer willpower needed to maintain the posture and perform the movements, my muscles went into even more violent spasms.

I couldn't even control my tongue movements. I frequently bit down on my tongue accidentally while eating, causing blood to pour out of my mouth. Then I'd unintentionally bite the swollen tongue again, so it never healed. Eventually, strange muscles of different colorations appeared on my tongue sheath. It progressively became more uncomfortable to talk as my sentences became slurred and my tongue and chin felt dull as if something was binding them together. Speaking itself became more difficult, and being aware of these symptoms, I became increasingly reluctant to talk.

My head, neck, and chin shook and pulsated, making it difficult to close my mouth and sip water. When my neck muscles moved uncontrollably, making it hard to swallow liquids, I had to use a straw. Thankfully, my daughter purchased a number of big, supple silicone straws. I used one to sip water and the other to take my herbal medicine.

I Can't Even Shampoo or Brush My Teeth by Myself

MEANWHILE, I LOST FEELING IN my fingertips. It started with just the index finger. One by one, the other fingers began to stiffen until all of the fingers on both hands lost their ability to move. In addition to eating and drinking, it was difficult to carry out basic hygiene tasks. Because I couldn't wash my own face properly, my daughter would use Eau de toilette to clean my face and then apply lotion.

But whereas other tasks were more or less manageable with help, cleaning my teeth was a different matter.

When my husband attempted to assist me with brushing my teeth one day, it didn't go well, so I tried to do it on my own. My movements were robotic and it was impossible to manage with the toothbrush because my jaw and mouth twisted up and froze.

My facial expression when I caught a glimpse of myself in the mirror was so peculiar that I wondered, "Who's that in the mirror?" Without realizing it, I had been grimacing like a fiend as I expended great effort for the task. I choked as I attempted to open my mouth as wide as possible and insert the toothbrush to brush my back teeth.

I made every effort to brush quickly. There was a lot of foam and saliva in my mouth and I couldn't breathe, especially as my panic level rose. I struggled, unsure of what to do. With a sharp gasp, I let out a breath.

My husband quickly helped me rinse out my mouth and lie down. An intense muscle contraction seemed to be taking place in my neck and shoulders. The tightening temporarily subsided as my husband pulled at my hands and extended my arms, but it was an ordeal that day trying to recover from the strain.

"Breathe out, relax your mind, breathe out, relax . . . "

My husband repeated the words as he tugged at my hands and shifted my arm positions. But it hardly made a difference.

I burst into tears. There was nothing I could do in the circumstance. I found that crying helped me breathe more easily and gave my mind a little relief. My husband dried my tears and consoled me. "Don't worry. I'm here by your side. I'll always be here. The difficult times will pass eventually."

I was unable to perform even routine everyday tasks like brushing my teeth without breathing problems. After this occurred several times, my husband declared he'd do everything for me himself.

Taking a shower was equally tough for me because my fingers were paralyzed and my right arm couldn't be lifted. My husband promised he'd wash my hair. He did a good job, but I didn't like having someone else do that for me.

One day, he shampooed my hair and used the shower wand to rinse it, but bubbles ended up getting in my ears, nose, and eyes. My eyes began to hurt.

"I'd much prefer the shower head!"

My husband did as I asked. I was prepared to just let it go and move on, but my husband suggested I lather up my hair again. I yelled.

"No, I got all the shampoo in my eyes!"

"You have to do it twice to get clean."

"No way! I won't do it two times. I can't open my eyes."

My husband was just trying to be nice to me, but instead of thanking him, I snapped at him. He must have felt embarrassed and disappointed to see me reacting in that way. My bad mood exacerbated my neck and back pain. There was no way to tell what worse things were in store.

My husband must have been rather displeased but he tugged on my hands and helped swing my arms back and forth to relieve them.

"You need to calm your mind. Anxiety can affect your body negatively."

I'm aware that sometimes I can be overly sensitive. I don't know how I got to be such a stubborn and angry "director-in-chief"!

In any case, having someone else shampoo my hair was, to put it mildly, difficult to handle. On days when I didn't shampoo and only showered, I turned on the shower tap and stood still under the stream. My husband would use a big towel to dry off my body after the shower and wrap it around me, and then I'd sprawl out on the bed. I missed my old, routine daily life so much, I wanted to cry.

My Senses Do a Sword Dance

MY HUSBAND SUGGESTED THAT I take a bath since it was hard for me to shower. He reasoned that immersing in warm water would help me feel better and loosen up my stiff body, and there was no need to stand up. He said that shampooing could be done on the spot and it would be much more convenient, so I agreed.

One day, my husband drew water in the tub and told me to get in.

But the moment I put one foot in the water, it felt so hot, I screamed.

"Ah! Ah! That's hot! What are you doing? It's way too hot."

I sobbed aloud as I stood in the bathtub, startled and afraid, not wanting to stay but unable to get out. Even without any of the normal triggers, my chin and neck began to convulse. When my already overheated body contacted the hot water, I thought I would lose it. I yelled to my husband to get me out of there immediately as he hastily turned on the cold water faucet.

"Uh, I didn't make it that hot . . . "

Saying these words, my husband hurriedly rescued me from the tub.

"My body isn't normal!"

My husband appeared to be as shocked as I was. I was afraid after that, and didn't take a bath again for some time.

My body was out of my control. Whenever someone washed me and applied lotion to my body, I often recalled my own mother, who battled high blood pressure and twice completely lost consciousness as a result.

She was still able to walk after her first collapse and continued with certain aspects of her daily routine after her release from the hospital. But after her second fall, she remained unwell and unable to get out of bed. It was what's known as a "cerebrovascular accident", also known as a stroke.

What I still can recall is how much my mother used to enjoy getting bathed by me. Although her daughter-in-law took consummate care of her and lived with her, mom appeared more at ease when her daughter helped her with her bath. She grinned and seemed so happy. How did she feel when she was unable to control her body and needed other hands to help her bathe? Now I knew. It's a pity that I wasn't able to help her more often.

There were some scary moments that are difficult to think back on. A few months prior to mom's passing, one of her arms began shaking violently while she was unconscious. When I said "Mom, mom", there was no response, just the shaking arm. It hurts so much that I was powerless to help her.

When I thought of the present me, lying immobilized, my arms and legs swaying randomly in the air, suspended from rubber straps attached to a structure installed in my bedroom, I realized how like my mother I was. It felt eerie and terrifying at the same time. I remembered that she'd forewarned me of this. The herbalist, after checking my pulse, had also warned me to be especially careful about constipation, saying that my blood was turbid, and that I was prone to developing palsy.

I'd lie down after taking a shower while my daughter or husband dressed me and lotioned my face and body. Just getting through each day was really challenging for me—challenging to send texts by cell phone, to make calls, to take pictures, and to type.

A Huntington Genetic Test and Cerebrospinal Fluid Test

"My body was like an oven and my skin broke out in sweats trying to cool down, even if I wasn't moving around."

Could There Be a Genetic Factor or Is It a Brain Problem?

MATTERS WERE GETTING WORSE. AFTER seeing how strangely my symptoms developed, my husband became more involved in my care. He emailed Prof. Park on August 1 and then visited Dongguk University Hospital the following day to pick up my new prescription. I was in no condition to accompany him. My husband's email from August 1 makes it quite evident that my condition was deteriorating at the time:

> *"There is one thing I want to ask you, which is why I am emailing you today. The patient's neck is stiff, particularly on the right side, and her right shoulder quakes and feels heavy, making it difficult for her to sit or use her hands. As a result, the patient's family is assisting her with meals.*
>
> *She lies down the majority of the time. But even then, she constantly swings her arms and legs from side to side. She sweats profusely as a result of the strong uncontrollable action of her muscles, therefore I would say she is*

getting a lot of exercise. So we're pursuing medication as a means to recovery. Yet, from the perspective of daily living, I wonder if there might be a method to ameliorate her difficult situation, described above. I am exploring several approaches, such as breathing exercises.

The specific concern I'm emailing you about today has to do with the patient's sleep. Currently, she takes one Alpram every evening. Sometimes the medication doesn't work, however, leaving her with no choice but to wait till enough time has passed to take another tablet and fall asleep. If you have any recommendations for the patient's sleep issue, please let me know. For instance, would taking two Alpram tablets when necessary be preferable to taking another medication, such as so-called "sleeping pills", along with it? As you are the expert who is caring for the patient, I'm writing to ask you."

Yet, there was no new solution. Her new guidance was to continue taking the previously prescribed medications as usual, but to take Alpram three times a day, at breakfast, lunch, and dinner; Rivotril in the evening; and Rivotril again at night if I had trouble falling asleep.

After seeing Prof. Park two weeks prior on the evening of July 16, my husband, who was still quite worried, emailed Prof. Jeon Beomseok. He gave Prof. Jeon an update on the situation and inquired about moving the treatment scheduled for September 11 to an earlier date.

My husband promised that we would follow Prof. Park's recommendations and continue to see her for treatment. However, he pointed out that during the month and a half of treatment from early June to mid-July, my condition had appeared to grow worse and there had been a lot of agony. He pointed to my experience on July 16, when I went from our home in Gangnam, Seoul to the hospital in Ilsan for an appointment, resting flat on my back in a comfortable car, yet it had been a significant strain. When I got home, I had to lie down and was unable to eat dinner.

My neck and upper back were so stiff that I couldn't sit down, he continued, and it was hard for me to eat and drink. He also mentioned that my neck muscles jerked erratically.

Because of this, he explained, he wanted to let Prof. Jeon know about my current worsening state and give him another chance to weigh in on any potential future actions. He also included a brief video that showed the strange pulsations in my neck.

Prof. Jeon then replied to us, stating that while he couldn't address my issues by email due to an eye operation he himself was having and the commencement of a new international project, he could arrange for a few exploratory tests.

So I saw Prof. Jeon on July 29. At the appointment, my husband presented the doctor with a summary he had produced of the therapy up to that point.

> "Since May 29, she has received four treatments ordered and administered by Prof. Park of Dongguk University Ilsan Hospital. Her next scheduled treatment is on September 17, 2019. The prescription medicines she

takes are Alpram, Lexapro, and Rivotril. In response to the patient's complaint that her condition is worsening, Prof. Park mentioned the possibility of performing a Huntington genetic test.

The biggest inconvenience the patient feels is that her neck is so stiff and sore that it is difficult to sit, stand, and walk, and that it is difficult to eat and brush her teeth. So she spends a lot of time lying down.

In addition to Prof. Park's treatments, she has joined a program three times a week to relieve her tension through breathing exercises. Also, a massage and acupressure specialist comes to our home at 8:30 pm, and my wife receives a massage for about an hour and a half."

On August 5, the Seoul National University Hospital performed a Huntington's genetic test by Prof. Jeon's order. He also requested that I undergo an autoimmune spinal fluid test while I was there. I went to get the spinal fluid extracted in the morning, waited for 7-8 hours until 4:00 pm, and then went home. The test results showed no evidence of a problem.

As mentioned earlier, the symptoms worsened from the end of June to the middle of July, and as summer temperatures began to rise, they grew worse still. I wasn't even trying to exercise because of my muscle tremors, since even when I was motionless, my body produced heat. Enduring the feverishness was no picnic. I had to run the air conditioner in my room all day long, it was so hot in and out. Everyone grumbled about how cold the room was. In fact, my limbs were as cold as ice. It was bizarre: my body was cold, but at the same time, I was panting from the heat.

My husband had built a tension relief structure in our bedroom, and one time, he entered the room and found me lying on the floor with my arms and legs in rubber straps. He approached and was about to pat me on the shoulder.

"Darling, you must be having a tough time."

Like a shot, I shouted at him,

"Ugh, it's hot! Go away!"

His hand brushing against my skin felt like fire. How awkward for my husband! We used to avoid using the A/C, even in the midsummer, because we hated the icy blasts of air. Yet, things were totally different now. My body was like an oven and my skin broke out in sweats trying to cool down, even if I wasn't moving around. My husband and daughter gave me their whole attention during the trying months of July and August. I clung to my husband like a baby as my condition deteriorated, and I grew anxious without him. My husband didn't even leave the house for work; he stayed home. He took care of me every day, from morning to night.

Are Drugs a Cure or an Addiction?

M Y TREATMENT CONTINUED AFTER MY movement disorder syndrome diagnosis without the use of any other medical intervention beyond medication. Although they are symptomatic therapies, acupressure, yoga, meditation, and massage haven't been well studied or proven to have any genuine health benefits. I tried everything I believed would be helpful. I was willing to grab at straws, but I never noticed any tangible positive impact.

At breakfast, lunch, and dinner, I took my prescribed prescriptions as well as a herbal supplement that was supposed to be healthy for the body. I was prescribed antidepressants and medications for panic disorder. They had a calming influence on my body, reducing the intensity of my trembling muscles and allowing me to wind down. When my body relaxed, my muscles could also relax and I could drift off to sleep.

On the other hand, the coercive function of the medications had a side-effect. I used to get sleepy after eating breakfast and taking my medications, so I'd go back to bed, then get up again, eat lunch, take my medications one more time, and take a nap. Dinner, more medications, and then another nap followed. In some ways, induced sleep aggravated my insomnia. I got to the point where even the medications weren't helping me sleep.

I spent the majority of the day drowsy from sleep, just lying in bed. My physical strength eventually declined owing to the vicious cycle this daily routine set in motion. Being confined to bed all day caused my energy levels to drop, my muscles to atrophy, and my activity to decline. Walking became more and more of a challenge as I lay on my back with my limbs suspended in rubber straps from the structure set up in our bedroom. In addition, I had to use a walker, which also caused my muscles to weaken.

Like many other patients, I had low motivation worsened by anxiety and depression, and there were also moments when the medications caused me to become lethargic and lose focus. I afterwards suffered the addition of dizziness.

My digestive tract was also acting strangely. I experienced long bouts of terrible constipation, intermittent diarrhea, and constant mouth dryness despite drinking plenty of water. This was caused in part by the intense sweating brought on by the uncontrollable body tremors. I had to bring water with me wherever I went, my mouth was so parched. I drank so much water, it made it hard to stay asleep because I had to get up frequently during the night.

Nonetheless, as sick as I was, I still had a strong appetite and ate better than one might suppose. But, strangely enough, I rapidly dropped weight. I lost so much weight that I yearned for the days when I believed I was overweight and had dieting on my list of things to do.

There appeared to be positive aspects on the one hand, and negative ones on the other, as my body completely lost its equilibrium. But I was unable to escape my predicament.

In this way I overcame my functional movement disorder syndrome, experiencing both the good effects and the bad side effects of the pharmacological therapy.

Oh, My Life is Over!

"Don't panic. You're fine. Let's try it again."
"Mom, you'll be OK, I promise."

An Emergency Pager Installed
Due to Shortness of Breath

S UDDEN SHORTNESS OF BREATH! EVEN when exercising vigorously, I'd never experienced breathing problems. Now, however,
I frequently found myself gasping for oxygen in the evenings when
my neck and back were convulsing severely. No one was choking
me, of course. But every time I felt like I was suffocating, the
anxiety was next to intolerable. Before, when I exercised beyond
my physical limit, breathing might have been harder than usual,
but now I was actually experiencing emergencies.

It was August 15. I was looking out the window. The weather
was cool and it was raining.

"Today I want to go outside!"

They were like the magic words my husband had been waiting
for; he was so happy. After lunch, it was still sprinkling, but my
husband led me outside to the yard, umbrella in tow.

"Look at the blossoms. So lovely!"

We strolled through the garden before stopping at Cloud Cafe
for a cup of tea. Because sitting was so painful, I stayed standing.
Despite some slight trembling, it was lovely.

Then we came home, where I fell asleep. When I woke up, my body was convulsing more violently than before for some reason. When I tried standing, my head went dizzy and my stomach went woozy. My husband and daughter helped me perform stretches that aided in reducing the tremors.

After finishing dinner, I tried sitting in the massage chair to relieve my sore neck and shoulders.

The machine massaged my upper and lower back and put pressure on my neck, causing my entire body to vibrate as it did. Although I made every effort to relax, the stimulation was too intense. I stayed with it for as long as I could, enduring the discomfort; but after a short while, I gave up and went straight to bed. In an effort to help me calm down, my husband grabbed both of my hands and tugged on them. Then he went to the kitchen to mix some vitamins. It was at that point that the convulsions really started to worsen.

"Argh! Ugh! Daughter, are you there? Darling!"

My throat constricted, choking me, before I could even yell to my daughter what was wrong.

My husband came running. My daughter, who was in the shower, also sprinted in, perplexed. My husband and daughter tried to calm my body down by pulling my arms over my head, extending and stretching them as far as they could, and caressing them, as well as my legs.

"Try exhaling. Come on! Hoo—, hoo—"

I tried to breathe but didn't have much success. I twisted and flailed in what must have seemed like utter anguish, as if I were suffocating. It was useless. Not knowing what to do, I burst out bawling.

"Don't panic. You're fine. Let's try it again."

"Mom, you'll be OK, I promise."

My daughter and husband spent a lot of time soothing, reassuring, and helping me breathe.

At the point of bursting into tears, I was able to breathe a little easier. What if there had been no one nearby or at home to come aid me?

When I was truly unable to breathe, or even when I just couldn't speak clearly, I thought, "My life is finished", but I also questioned why I was being subjected to the agony. What major sin have I committed to deserve this? I wondered. To be honest, when the thought of dying crossed my mind, I'd break down. At such times, I'd sob uncontrollably while holding my husband close.

If someone had asked me then when I was happiest, I'd have said, "When I'm asleep". I yearned to flee the suffering. It was better for me just sleep since that way, I had nothing to worry about or think about.

Now, leaving me in the room alone was a cause for concern. After much deliberation, the family opted to buy and install a pager. Due to his work schedule, my husband was unable to be by my side at all times during the day. My daughter, who owns a private business, took turns with my husband looking after me.

I lay all day on a mat spread out in front of the bed, with my arms and legs in rubber straps. I had to ask someone for help whenever I wanted to get a drink of water or use the restroom. It was difficult to yell and it was difficult to get up and ask for help, so we placed the pager in a spot that was easy to reach, next to the bed.

I had the pager set up to buzz in my daughter's room when pressed. I put another one in the restroom. That way, my daughter could come and help me in an emergency. There was already a rope in the bathroom I could hold, to support me when standing up.

Is This Really the End?: A Time of Despair Begins

THINGS APPEARED TO HAVE REACHED a point of near hopelessness as daily tasks got harder and breathing started to become a regular battle. Even attending gatherings and meetings with my friends was no longer possible. My friends started to worry when they heard I was sick and started to phone and message me.

But I didn't always pick up the phone. Actually, I couldn't. Not only could I not pick up the phone, I also had no idea what to say. Some of my friends expressed their feelings through texts when I didn't answer their calls. These brief phone calls and messages were very consoling.

Questions like "How's your health?" were texted by those who were unaware of how serious my physical situation was, while friends who were fully aware called to offer their support. I just replied, "It's still up and down". I couldn't think of anything else to say.

"Young-hee, I was shocked to hear the news. I called you but you didn't pick up. If the hospital doesn't know

how to treat it, you'll have to look elsewhere. How about asking someone who's skilled in using pulse reading to identify diseases, or someone who's good at acupuncture, etc.? If you take positive action with hope and courage, good results will come. Get better quickly, I'll see you later and we'll have a fun time then."
—College friend 1 (2019. 6. 27.)

"I'm in Gapyeong. The weather's nice and cool here. I wake up in the morning and think of you. I've been thinking of you since last week. I wonder how you're doing . . . "
—College friend 2 (2019. 7. 23.)

"Young-hee! How are you doing these days?"
—College friend 3 (2019. 8. 24.)

"I hope you're getting better. Isn't there a famous doctor somewhere you can contact? Actually, I was reminded of a TV program I saw in Japan. Isn't there a doctor in Japan who can help you find the cause of your symptoms?"
—College friend 3 (2019. 8. 24.)

A college friend who heard that I had to eat with my left hand because I couldn't lift my right arm, told me about an easy-to-eat spoon for the disabled, and suggested I try it.

"Young-hee, I will pray hard for you. Where there's a will, there's a way. It's summer weather now, so eat a lot of nutritious food, get plenty of rest, and only think about good things . . . "
—High school friend 1 (2019. 8. 9.)

"You're not picking up. I called because they said you were taking calls. I'm worried but I don't want to bother you . . . If it's okay with you, I'd love to see you in person . . . I wish I could call you . . . is there a convenient time for me to stop by, or is this an unreasonable request? It's okay if you don't reply. I am always praying for your speedy recovery."
—High school friend 2 (2019. 10. 2.)

Another friend revealed to me that she was visiting her husband who was a patient at Samsung Hospital. To commemorate the hospital's 25th anniversary, there was a "Make-a-Wish" event. She said she had inscribed the following wish on a green ball:

"I wish for Shim Young-hee's recovery."
—High school friend 3 (2019. 12. 18.)

A friend of mine who graduated from the same department and went on to become a professor called me one day. She called me once on June 15 and again on August 23. My symptoms started to appear in June, and the worst stretch of the disease was in August. Which of those two times it was, I'm not sure.

As I was unwell, it was difficult for me to pick up my cell phone. I used a speakerphone to answer her call. Oddly, despite being sick, my voice got louder.

Maybe it was to mask the discomfort. Things were complicated in my head, but I probably pretended to be upbeat on the outside. But I found it difficult to keep my emotions fully hidden. I discovered that I was sharing my heart with her as we chatted about this and that.

"I believed my life was over . . . I was a sobbing mess."

But, even then, I put on a cool exterior as if I were discussing past history. My heart ached so badly that I wept silently after hanging up the phone.

I questioned whether my life had truly ended.

A New Movement Disorder Pattern:
What Should I Do Now?

"I tried to raise my arm, but it felt leaden and stayed rooted to the spot, as if I were attempting to lift a massive iron weight."

From Muscle Tremors to Hardness and Stiffness

I DON'T KNOW WHEN HE STARTED, but my husband always kept notes about my condition and home recovery in preparation for the next medical checkup. This helped me and the other family members, and also offered lateral support by giving the medical team accurate information about my progress during the extremely brief treatment times.

Needless to say, average treatment time per patient at large hospitals in Korea, only two to three minutes at most, is insufficient. Moreover, patients like me, who are undergoing long-term treatment and who don't see noticeable changes right away, are treated very infrequently, at intervals of one or two months or more. As such, it's difficult for the so-called "attending physician" to even remember the patient: all he or she has to do is scan the medical data right before meeting them. It's a structure in which the patient must be the one to take the initiative, to actively ask for something.

On September 11, 2019, I went to Seoul National University Hospital for an appointment with Prof. Jeon.

After my initial appointment on May 20, I underwent testing while hospitalized from May 26 to May 30. On August 5, the spinal fluid and Huntington's genetic tests were performed, followed by a meeting with the doctor to discuss the results. When we arrived to my appointment, the doctor read the notes my husband had brought with him and learned about my physical condition up to that point.

The notes included an overview of my deteriorating health, the challenges I faced every day, and my current pharmaceutical regimen.

Above all, the notes stated that despite controlling the amount of food I ate, my weight had drastically fallen and was now under 50 kg. The notes also indicated that all ten of my fingers had some degree of paralysis and that my left index finger had weakened, wouldn't flex, and was basically useless.

Regarding daily challenges, the notes pointed out that I had to eat soft foods and that chewing food, in particular, was a big hurdle. The washing and patting techniques I used to wash my face and clean my teeth were also harder to do.

The notes informed Prof. Jeon that I'd doubled my Lexapro dosage, that I was taking 0.5 mg of Alpram twice a day, once in the morning and once in the evening, and one Rivotril tablet in the morning but not in the evening. I also had to take an extra dose of Rivotril if the Alpram I took in the evening didn't put me to sleep.

I was asked to raise my arm during the exam by the resident standing next to Prof. Jeon, but I couldn't do it. The only thing I could move was my hand; the arm wouldn't budge. On May 20, when I first visited the hospital, my arm had been fully functional. I was able to raise it, rotate my hand, and open and close a fist.

"The pattern has changed."

Prof. Jeon noted that what began as the main symptom, the muscle tremors, was the lesser issue now. He noted that my right arm was rigid and wouldn't move, and that as a result, I was showing signs of an abnormal gait.

When Prof. Jeon asked me if I was receiving physical therapy at Ilsan Hospital, I told him that I was on medications and nothing else. He replied that in that case, it wasn't necessary to spend effort traveling so far. He mentioned that he was working jointly with another professor at Seoul National University Hospital. If I chose to switch physicians, he'd make arrangements for me to get treatment from him. I expressed my desire to switch doctors. He scheduled an appointment for me with Professor Ham Bong-jin of the psychiatry division. Then we left.

That day, my husband and daughter-in-law went with me to the hospital. While we waited for about thirty minutes, my daughter-in-law supported my right arm with her own, just like my husband always did. She appeared the next day with her neck and shoulder covered in Icy Hot patches. Heavens, I thought, my right arm must have been heavy. I really felt bad about it.

My Inability to Lift My Right Arm or Walk with a Normal Gait

I N THE INTERIM, SEOUL NATIONAL University Hospital provided me with a diagnosis and a prescription, and on September 17, as scheduled, I visited Prof. Park Jung E. One can understand how much my situation had changed by looking at the details that my husband, in consultation with me, had recorded at the time.

> *"The patient received a medical referral on May 29, 2019, from Prof. Jeon at Seoul National University Hospital, and on June 3, she saw Prof. Park for the first time. Her neck muscles were shaking, but she didn't find it difficult to sit, move, bathe, use the phone, or use the Internet on a daily basis. Her present state is poor compared to then. Above all, the patient's hands and arms remain by her sides and are virtually paralyzed. She is unable to perform tasks that involve using her hands, such as eating and brushing her teeth, or anything else that calls for hand strength, therefore she is quite dependent on her family.*
>
> *Thinking back, the patient's daily life was exceedingly challenging when I urgently phoned Prof. Park on August 1. Even with air conditioning, she couldn't sleep comfortably at night since she was constantly lying down and sweating profusely. But, she now has acquired a good bit of "know-how" and is managing to live a normal life with the support of her family.*

The tremor in her arms, particularly her right arm, is, nonetheless, very pronounced. It is not merely quivering; sometimes there is the very powerful push-and-pull of muscular spasms. The patient has no idea how much stress is being exerted on her arm. Instead, she complains about her sore neck, the strain on her shoulders, and difficulty getting around with her arm frozen at her side. Notably, she finds it difficult to leave her right hand alone because it always needs to be grasping something. With the assistance of her family, she can now stand and walk, but she still finds it very difficult to sit in a chair.

She saw Prof. Jeon in his office on September 11, and he informed her that the autoimmune and genetic tests for Huntington's disease that Prof. Park had discussed had all come out negative. He declared that "the pattern has changed" after observing the patient's gait and bodily movements. When he inquired about Prof. Park's treatment plan, we replied that my wife was taking her medication as directed. He also asked whether she was receiving physical therapy."

While it was acknowledged that my physical health had improved, it was also obvious that my condition had changed. Even though the tremors in my neck and back had lessened, my right arm was rock-hard and I couldn't move it from my side, making it impossible to move naturally back and forth while walking.

I tried to raise my arm, but it felt leaden and stayed rooted to the spot, as if I were attempting to lift a massive iron weight.

Normally, walking involves switching one's weight from left to right automatically as one moves one's legs, but because my right arm was like granite, I constantly leaned to the left. My center of gravity would shift to one side, nearly toppling me over, and my right shoulder would hitch up at an awkward angle, resulting in a gait that was something between a waddle and a limp. I needed someone to physically support my right arm to help me walk.

In addition, my right arm was twisted out of shape, my right palm facing outward from my body instead of naturally descending down from shoulder to knee.

I was in an unusual and embarrassing situation that brought to mind the people with disabilities, such as Dr. Stephen Hawking, I'd seen on television. I'd look the same way, I thought.

I had no idea whom I was looking at in the mirror. I sensed that it wasn't me. I was afraid. My gaze seemed to be fixed on an infinite chasm.

What should I do now?

PART 2

. . .

It's Okay, I'm Here

CHAPTER 3

• • •

*The Wisdom to Find
the Best Solution*

Regret Cannot Erase
How Sorry I Feel

*"Your mother may not express it, but in her heart, she feels a lot of
anxiety and worry. It shouldn't ever be allowed to build up. Let's
all keep this in mind and treat your mother accordingly."*

It Took 50 Years to Realize

END OF MAY 2019. ACCORDING to Prof. Jeon at Seoul National
University Hospital:

"Stress is to blame. You've been a scholar your entire life.
You've faced and overcome a lot of stress. I have no idea why this
functional disorder has only started to appear now, but going
forward, you have to relearn everything, including how to breathe
and walk."

In fact, before meeting Prof. Jeon, I had assumed that my
wife Young-hee would always be by my side with her unwavering
intelligence and good health, as she was in the past. She had some
discomfort on the day of her diagnosis, but she had no issues with
sitting and standing, eating, or taking a shower.

But, the professor's statements seemed like a warning that far
worse things were yet to come. The future looked bleak.

From 2014 through 2018, we spent our summers in the southern French city of Aix-en-Provence. This is because Young-hee
and I had the good fortune to take part in a project funded by
the European Union. Before coming back to Korea in 2018, we

left our belongings with a French coworker and put a 500 euro deposit down on the flat where we lived, with the intention of returning to France again in 2019. I was saddened by Prof. Jeon's remarks as I faced the possibility that our plans might fall apart.

But as Young-hee's condition swiftly declined and her recuperation took precedence, my perspective completely shifted. I started to think about the various facets of her failing health that I had contributed to. I became angrier the more I reflected on the past; sometimes it was vehement remorse, and other times it felt like an unstoppable storm had assaulted and taken hold of me.

September 2018 is the first thing that came to mind. We took a train from Aix-en-Provence to Lyon for a seminar, stopped in Munich, Germany, where we met with friends, took the S-Bahn to Starnberg, where we saw Professor Habermas, and then took a flight back to Lyon. After boarding the TGV there, we returned to Aix-en-Provence about midnight. It was a very tight schedule and a tiring day for me, but even more so for Young-hee.

Young-hee suggested that we take a taxi because she was tired. The cost would be 50 euros. We also had two large suitcases. A large number of people left in cars parked in the station's parking lot, while others took taxis. There were very few people waiting for the bus. The bus we intended to catch, which left from the Marseille Airport, came only infrequently during the wee hours of the morning. We sat on the steps where people ascended to board the train and descended to board the bus, and waited. But the bus did not come for quite some time. Young-hee was worn out.

"I'm exhausted. I'm dead! Let's take a taxi!"

Young-hee was drooping like a wet sock as she crouched down and leaned against her suitcase.

A respectable husband would have hailed a taxi. But despite Young-hee's admonishments, I disregarded the idea. It wasn't that we lacked the money. It was because I was stuck stubbornly in my belief that taking a taxi was a waste of cash. After a long wait, we finally boarded a bus headed to the city of Aix-en-Provence, where we eventually arrived at our accommodations, lugging our bulky baggage.

I was unaware of my fault at the time. Later, however, as Young-hee's health declined and I discovered that stress was to blame, this recollection morphed into a mirror that revealed this incredibly terrible part of myself that was dogmatic, cold-hearted, and one-sided. As the scene rushed back to me, calling me an "idiot!", it lashed at my conscience mercilessly.

"You idiot! Why do you focus on yourself so much in everything you do?"

"Why did you show such disregard for your wife's excruciating fatigue?"

"What did that accomplish for you? What did you achieve?"

Looking back, I realize that I ignored Young-hee's exhaustion up until May 2019. I frequently invited international academics as part of the Joongmin Foundation's activities, such as John Dunn from the University of Cambridge in the U.K., Scott Lash from Oxford University, and Professor Zhang Jing from Beijing University.

Young-hee was there at each and every one of these occasions. The schedules were also quite tight. There were regional gatherings in Gwangju and Jeonju, numerous seminars in Seoul, and protracted afterparties. Young-hee was quite fatigued at the time since she was already displaying early signs of a mobility issue. She repeatedly told me she wanted to go home, but I persisted in being a disinterested husband. I should never have done that, ever.

I was also aware early on that Young-hee had trouble falling asleep. Yet I didn't see it as a problem of mine. I believed that sleep was a personal issue, a thing that nobody else could help with.

When the French book *La dynastie rouge*, which details the three generations of North Korea's ruling family, was translated and published by Joongmin Publishers, Young-hee proofread and revised the translation. At times she worked until late at night because she couldn't sleep, and other times she woke up in the middle of the night and continued working until morning. I tried to get her to ease up a little, because I was concerned that she had to do all that work, but there was nothing I could do to stop her. I never considered that maybe there was something I could have done to help Young-hee sleep comfortably.

Later, as Young-hee's condition deteriorated, I made the decision to live by the mantra, "Help Young-hee get to sleep first, then I can sleep." I quickly discovered that Young-hee was able to enter dreamland more easily with my help. That's when I first realized that I could have taken action long ago to address Young-hee's insomnia, had I recognized it as an issue for me as well. Her sleeping problem had not bothered me because I assumed it was a personal issue and had nothing to do with me.

I didn't understand that my indifference, short-sightedness, and egocentric thinking were the fundamental causes of the problem, until Young-hee fell ill. I was also able to feel the depth of a husband and wife's physical and mental rapport more clearly.

I had not recognized it in 50 years of marriage . . .

Things the Family Should Do for Mom's Health

THE FIRST THING I NEEDED to do as Young-hee's movement disorder steadily worsened was to ensure that everyone stay patient and cooperative while also keeping the family informed about the disease's etiology and available treatments. What the family was witnessing was a type of muscle spasm, aberrant movement in Young-hee's neck muscles, of an unknown origin.

Understandably, different viewpoints were expressed. Thus, on July 22, I sent an email to our daughter, son, and his wife summarizing the course of treatment over the preceding few months:

> "A professor at Seoul National University Hospital Gangnam Center treated your mother for her neck tremors and other health problems in February [2019]. He said that no irregularities could be observed in the MRA data. Her symptoms grew worse, though. On May 20, Prof. Jeon Beomseok, from the same hospital, began treating your mother.
>
> Prof. Jeon said he discovered no structural anomalies. Nonetheless, since the symptoms persisted, he recommended that she consult Prof. Park at Dongguk University Ilsan Hospital. She began taking the Alpram Prof. Park

had prescribed on June 4. It has been roughly 50 days as of today, July 22.

It is accurate to say that her current state of health is worse than it was in the past. She was in a lot of pain when she had her initial checkup with Prof. Park on June 3, but she had no significant issues with walking, standing, or sitting. While standing has been more comfortable for her than sitting, she now finds it difficult to walk. She also finds it difficult to sit. Her hands do not move the way she wants them to and she cannot move freely due to the stiffness in the back of her neck. In these situations, it's usually beneficial to learn about our alternatives for the future from a number of sources. We also want to talk amongst ourselves about how we can support your mother.

... However, it appears that expecting a neat causal factor analysis, or hoping for a complete recovery in a short period of time, is not realistic. It is a condition that is difficult to define using current disease nomenclature, and is part of an ambiguous disease terrain characterized by a common symptom, namely, involuntary muscle movement. On June 18, at the second session, Prof. Park prescribed Lexapro, which she anticipated would start working after six weeks. It would take about a year to complete the treatment, she said.

Recently, she has experienced less activity in her neck muscles when she is lying down. A new symptom, soreness and stiffness in her neck, makes it difficult to walk. A basic course of treatment is being administered in accordance with the good and dependable doctor's prescription, and by combining our knowledge and resources, we hope to find a way to restore normalcy to your mother's daily life. Here are my opinions in this regard.

. . . Never say or even imply that you are afraid or anxious about the future in front of your mother. Let's make a concerted effort to convey to her a message of hope and optimism that recalls happy memories and looks forward to more of those happy experiences once she recovers. The truth is that experts like Prof. Jeon, Prof. Park, and the Director of BATAE have determined that your mother is a patient who has a "psychological" ailment. This means that your mother's psychology and mind are both at the root of her condition and the solution to curing it. Your mother may not express it, but in her heart, she feels a lot of anxiety and worry. It shouldn't ever be allowed to build up. Let's all keep this in mind and treat your mother accordingly.

In addition to the neck muscle activity, the back of her neck is now so stiff that it is challenging for her to sit and walk. She seems to feel more at ease while lying down, but if this condition persists, there is a significant chance of more negative effects. We must therefore work to help her in moving her body organically, which will mean exerting a great deal of willpower.

The rehabilitation program run by Gangnam St. Mary's Hospital and the physical therapy provided by "BATAE" are crucial in this regard. More essential, *keep expanding on what you learn at home, to the extent that her body permits. You should not leave it up to your mom alone. We are all expected to exercise wisdom and work closely together."*

The Sadness of Watching Her Suffer

"Don't you worry. In time, it will seem like this never happened.
You have a son, a daughter-in-law, a daughter, and me,
all by your side. Try to keep a peaceful frame of mind."

Living Day-to-Day

THE LARGEST DIFFICULTY AROSE WHILE accompanying Young-hee on her daily walks.

Today, July 21, we were outside with our grandchildren at Banpo Stadium. Young-hee was walking behind the kids. She was having fun, keeping an eye on them and calling out their names as they ran around. Now, though, going outside is more difficult for her. We took a little stroll and she did some stretching, but it was tough for her because her neck was sore.

When Young-hee arrived back at the apartment, she promptly fell asleep. Even though she had only spent a short while walking around on a cool, windy day, I noticed that she was covered in perspiration when I helped her change into her bedclothes.

"I can barely walk. Aren't you frustrated?"

"Why say that? You do your best."

Young-hee was an excellent walker, in fact. She had enjoyed taking walks up until recently, and I had urged her to continue taking them. But things are different now. She finds it challenging to move around with her sore neck. Even waving her hand back and forth is difficult.

"My body doesn't move the way it should. Will I ever fully recover?"

"The doctor said that it would take a year."

"Yet, things just keep getting worse . . ."

A tinge of melancholy could be heard in the words. I assured her that we would beat the illness, in time.

"Yes, compared to the past, it's worse. But the illness has a course that it must run. Even with medication, you won't feel better immediately. There will be good and bad days. Besides, your neck tremor seems to have eased a little."

"The stiffness is a bigger problem than the tremors."

"We need to find out whether the stiffness is caused by the movement disorder or whether there are other causes. The masseur worked so hard to relax your neck. We need to look further into the question of whether your discomfort when sitting has anything to do with your neck muscles."

As dusk fell, our daughter-in-law arrived and fixed a meal of lettuce wraps and tender roast beef. She also made a broth that tasted like a smooth oxbone soup. After my son, his wife, and I had finished our meal, I helped Young-hee eat. She perspires during meals, but not as much during the evening. She had some melon and grapes for dessert. After supper, Young-hee went to sleep. She needed a rest.

Young-hee tried sitting against the bed, her legs on the floor, then tried lying stretched forward, but she was unable to find a position that was comfortable. It was bedtime. She lay down on the mattress after taking one Alpram.

"Don't you worry. In time, it will seem like this never happened. You have a son, a daughter-in-law, a daughter, and me, all by your side. Try to keep a peaceful frame of mind."

Young-hee said something sudden and unexpected.

"I must have committed many sins."

"Yet, Christianity, particularly Catholicism, sees suffering as having a purpose . . . as a process, of having one's sins washed away by suffering, then atoning for the sins of the entire world. Through suffering, you feel that your heart is being purified and that you are approaching salvation. Devout Christians reflect on Jesus' sufferings."

"I have to endure this suffering in order to change."

A bright flash of light pierced Young-hee's words.

"Right, that's the solution. We hope that this experience will strengthen our family bonds and help you change and improve. Just relax and think positively."

Even after taking Alpram, Young-hee typically falls asleep after an hour of tossing and turning. Tonight was no different.

"What were you thinking about? Would you like some music on the radio?"

I turned on some soothing music, gave Young-hee a kiss, and said softly,

"Sleep well."

"Thank you." (7. 21.)

How to Solve Problems of the Mind

IT SEEMS I SLEPT IN a little later than usual this morning—something I had not done in a while. It was half past eight when I woke up. Young-hee had already taken her herbal medicine for the morning and taken a shower. She told me to get some more sleep.

"You still haven't had breakfast?"

I got out of bed, washed my face, and had some abalone porridge that was waiting on the stove for breakfast, along with some kimchi. I filled my bowl to the brim with porridge and ate it all. Later, after taking her medication, Young-hee left for Mapo to get a massage.

I helped Young-hee with lunch, and then I went to the Express Bus Terminal bookstore to buy a book on body stretches. Afterwards I visited "BATAE Studio", which is close to Nambu Terminal, and had a 30-minute consultation with the director there. We had an interesting conversation getting ready for Young-hee's first visit the following day.

After dinner, it was already too late to take Young-hee outside. I read her my letter to the children.

"It's a long letter."

I gave her my personal view of why experts like Prof. Jeon, Prof. Park, and the BATAE Director believed her condition to be "psychological" or a mental health issue.

"You should be tuning out a lot of things right now since you're unwell, yet you keep wanting to *tune in* . . ."

"E-mails, downloads, I can't do anything."

"Those are physically challenging. I'm talking about your feelings."

Young-hee constantly nagged me about having to do this, that, or the other.

"I'll leave for a bit, then come back. What time do you take your medication?"

"I'll take it on my own. There's plenty of water here."

I left around 10:00 pm, spent some time walking around the playground, and returned around 11:00 pm. Young-hee, watching TV, greeted me. After washing my face and removing my sweat-stained tee shirt, I was about to say something to her. But, Young-hee had fallen asleep. She had been waiting for me, and when she saw that I was back, immediately dropped off. (7. 22.)

"The Lord's Prayer" Song at Midnight

"Young-hee expressed disappointment and said she had entirely lost the urge to go to sleep. It was already 2:00 in the morning. I was upset. But there was nothing I could do to help . . ."

All I Can Do Is . . .

Young-hee was in good shape when she woke up. After lunch, I used the basement gym to work out and shower for the first time in a while. Young-hee was about to doze off on a mat on the floor when I returned, huddled under a thin blanket. The A/C unit was running. I covered her with a big blanket she asked me for. She eventually fell asleep.

Because she slept, I assumed Young-hee would be in a good state. She woke up and we had dinner, a wonderful treat of Chinese Sichuan cuisine that she hadn't eaten in many months. (If you don't pick off the peppers, the dish is very spicy.) Sure enough, Young-hee was panting heavily when I entered the room after dinner. She was not feeling well and her body was agitated and restless. She calmed down a little after drinking some water.

The masseur arrived with Mr. Kim, our driver. Although it was Sunday, I thought it would be beneficial to have him assess Young-hee's condition since her first massage earlier on Friday. This time, the massage was different. Young-hee requested a massage specifically for her stiff neck, so the masseur concentrated on her neck, shoulders, and back. Young-hee did not respond when the masseur repeatedly asked her if she was experiencing discomfort. When he asked if there was any pain, Young-hee responded "no".

"Most people feel pain when I massage them this hard, but you're not reacting. Strange."

The masseur claimed that while loosening up Young-hee's shoulders and neck, he had first worked on one side then switched to the other, back and forth, and that each time he changed sides, he found the same tension in the same spot he had worked on just moments earlier. That is how it appeared to me as well. I could see as I looked on that while he massaged the stiff, difficult-to-release muscles on the left, the muscles on the right exhibited a strong involuntary response, and vice-versa.

Young-hee declared at the end of the hour-and-a-half session that unlike the first massage, which she believed had relaxed her, this one had not. The masseur described Young-hee's situation as quite unusual and stated, before departing, that he was unsure whether he could be of further assistance to the patient. I took the long view and made the decision that Young-hee should have massages three times a week.

But, Young-hee had problems falling asleep after the massage. Her neck was tensing up a lot. I reassured her that if she took her medication, she would be able to fall asleep, and I had her take a pill. She was still unable to sleep.

Young-hee expressed disappointment and said she had entirely lost the urge to go to sleep. It was already 2:00 in the morning. I was upset. But there was nothing I could do to help, so I suggested she take another pill. Young-hee was in great pain and said "yes" immediately. Suddenly, out of the blue, she invited me to join her in a song. It never crossed my mind that she would ask me to do that.

We got out of bed and stood holding hands, then began singing "The Lord's Prayer". We sang it several times. I advised Young-hee to have some water since her throat was dry. I told her to just listen instead of singing, but anyway, we stood and sung it several times holding hands before going back to bed.

Young-hee said that my singing was making her emotional. She cried and kept crying hysterically for a time. I stroked her back and hair to make her feel better.

"What are you afraid of when you have me, your son, daughter-in-law, and daughter right here by your side?"

I sang "The Lord's Prayer" to Young-hee as she lay there. I sang for a long time.

"That's enough, now. I think I'm going to sleep."

"Fine, then. I'll be right outside."

I went to the study. I started drafting a recommendation letter for one of my international students. Young-hee was dozing when I returned to the room a while later. I finished the recommendation letter, sent it by email, switched off the A/C and electric fan, and went to bed. (7. 28.)

The Difference Between What Must Be Discarded and the Strength to Endure

YOUNG-HEE'S CONDITION THIS MORNING WASN'T as good as yesterday, maybe as a result of the issues last night. She slept for a short time. We had to leave the apartment at 10:30 am since her appointment with Prof. Jeon was moved to an earlier time, 11:30.

Right before noon, the Seoul National University Hospital was incredibly busy. There was nowhere to take a seat. When we arrived at 11:15, Young-hee was the final patient on Prof. Jeon's appointment list. We had to wait until after 1:00 to see him since there was a backlog of patients ahead of us.

Because of a recent eye surgery, Prof. Jeon's vision was blurry. He also had a cast on his left hand, so he was a patient himself. He offered us guidance on several matters and made a number of diagnoses. He arranged for a procedure to collect fluid from Young-hee's spinal cord to test for autoimmune deficiency, along with an additional test for the Huntington gene. He apologized, added that he ought to be serving us better, but that due to his health at the moment, he needed our understanding. I thanked him for responding to my latest email so quickly and kindly, despite his being busy and unwell. Blood was drawn promptly as ordered and the additional tests were scheduled for August 5.

By the time we completed everything and returned home, it was after 2:30. We had been at the hospital for over three hours. The unexpected thing was that Young-hee had not rested once during the entire time. This was a significant discovery because the same thing could not have happened at home.

I believe that what happened that day was a "happiness amid calamity", like witnessing a light in the shadows. It appeared as though our sincere prayers from the previous evening had been answered. It gave us wisdom.

We learned that Young-hee was able to bear her discomfort for more than three hours without lying down. I believed that if we carefully navigated the situation, one step at a time, we could eventually resolve her issues.

On that basis, I reasoned that Young-hee needed to reduce her tension, and things like a warm bath at night would help. It appeared to be the right course to take because the main problem was how to lessen the constriction in Young-hee's muscles.

Young-hee awoke at dinnertime after a long, sound sleep. When our daughter saw her mother slowly enter the dining room, she commented with a smile: "Mom looks like grandma today." Young-hee generally has a vibrant, youthful appearance, but tonight she looked exhausted. I threw in my two cents:

"Yes, mom needs to be exhausted and lose her strength more than anything right now. The first step in her healing is to do just that!"

Young-hee enjoyed her meal. She had fallen asleep right after lunch and woke up without any difficulty, and had good digestion and a hearty appetite.

Young-hee's neck and body were calm. That appeared to be the outcome of obtaining enough sleep. After watching TV for a while, a little after 9:00, I drew her bath water.

Young-hee agreed that having a bath would help her to relax. Afterwards, I added more hot water and had a long soak myself, something I had not done in what seemed like ages. While lying side by side in bed and watching TV, the two of us recapped what we had learned from our day's schedule and from Prof. Jeon's consultation. About an hour after she had taken her medication, I suggested,

"Wouldn't it be a good idea to get ready for bed now?"

"Then turn the TV off. Let's have some music on the radio."

Young-hee appeared ready to turn in for the evening.

"Would you like me to sing 'The Lord's Prayer' again tonight?"

"No, that's alright. Your throat will get sore."

"I worried about that, so I brewed some Pu-erh tea and brought it in a large cup."

"You really are kind."

I then sang "The Lord's Prayer" in a low voice. After singing it a few times, she said that was enough. While sipping the tea, I sung it numerous times again, softly.

Then it grew quiet. If Young-hee's body was still, it meant that she was asleep. Nevertheless, I sang it several times again.

Before leaving the room, I turned off the A/C and the fan. I have to sum up the process of the past few days, which is why I am writing this right now. God has, after all, endowed us with wisdom. That is, before looking for far-off solutions, one should consider what can be done here and now. I genuinely appreciate it and will always be thankful for it. (7. 29.)

Gradually Uncovering Life's Clues

"The breathing exercises were challenging. The techniques that practice "letting go" and emphasize emptying the mind, using the body."

Don't Hate Me!

I TOOK YOUNG-HEE TO THE COMMUNITY center before dinner, where we took our time strolling through the cool hallways. She stood or sat for more than three hours yesterday without lying down, and did well even after she came home.

I had hoped that we would be able to have a leisurely stroll for an hour or so, maybe sit down and have a conversation. She requested we leave after thirty minutes, though, so we did.

Under circumstances where she is powerless, Young-hee accepts everything with grace. That is how I see it. But she has a propensity to give up easily if any other option presents itself.

Because of yesterday's positive experience, Young-hee suggested taking another bath tonight after dinner. Similar to the last time, I drew warm water into the bathtub. But Young-hee yelled "Oww!" as soon as she dipped in her foot, complaining that it was too hot.

I was really baffled for a second. Young-hee was trembling as though in dread as I swiftly turned on the cold water. Without more ado, I left the bathroom with her and began trying to calm her down.

First, my mind went blank, then it went hazy. I was incredibly sorry for Young-hee. I need to closely monitor Young-hee's physical health and take appropriate action based on my observations, but I was caught off guard, preoccupied as I was with my own thoughts from yesterday.

Young-hee had trouble falling asleep, even at 12:30 am. I sang to her, helped her stretch her arms, and wiped off her perspiration, but sleep would not come. It would be better to take another pill, I said. Young-hee agreed.

"Your thinking is the most crucial issue. Put everything out of your mind, unwind, and sleep."

I kissed Young-hee on the cheek and told her good night. She then made another unexpected comment.

"Don't hate me."

"How could I hate you?"

"Earlier, I gave you such a shock."

"I'm to blame. How surprised you were! The sight of you trembling like that . . . whew. We're going to change the way we give you a bath starting tomorrow night."

Young-hee apologized for startling me.

I try to focus all my attention on Young-hee when I speak to her, but when I act, I often do so in a way that suits me and what I want. The same thing happened tonight. (7. 30.)

You're Not Alone

I MUST HAVE BEEN EXHAUSTED. I awoke after 9:00 am. The only medication remaining for Young-hee to take after finishing her breakfast and taking her herbal medicine was the one that calms her nerves. Our brunch was made by our daughter.

I got up, washed my face, and drank a sip of the fermented drink I have every day. Then we headed to the BATAE Studio, taking bottled water to drink on the way.

Our last meeting was five days ago. The director welcomed us and asked us how we were. Young-hee said that she wasn't feeling well. She said that although it wasn't easy, she was working on her breathing exercises at home. She also talked about what happened after the session with the masseur. She said that she wanted to practice her exercises at the studio for as long as possible. She exercised for nearly an hour and a half, much longer than she usually did. The director and trainer stayed with her, patiently asking questions, while diagnosing her condition and demonstrating the correct exercises and techniques.

The breathing exercises were challenging. The techniques that practice "letting go" and emphasize emptying the mind, using the body. Young-hee, however, lacks experience and training in entirely clearing her mind. She tends toward perfectionism, always has a lot of work to do, and is always aware of her surroundings.

Some of the new information we learned today I will note down.

First of all, Young-hee should talk and sing more. She can wind down by talking a lot about other people, happy memories, etc. instead of focusing on herself.

A little walking is also beneficial. She should lightly bounce her shoulders as she walks. The neck muscles may suffer bad effects from forceful acupressure, which is dangerous and must be avoided. For her, it is crucial to relax—to let out her tension.

A 'half body soak' is also beneficial. For her neck, a cold-steamed pad would be helpful, and for the stomach, a warm pad. Her neck is hot and gets sweaty. The abdomen contains core muscles that, when tightened, can be massaged and loosen with heat. She shouldn't use cold steam on her neck if she has a bad reaction.

She should also gently rotate her shoulders up and down to exercise them. She needs to do movements that help release tension.

Her body appeared to loosen up at BATAE; but when she returned home, there were no indications that anything had significantly changed. She began meditating with our son after lunch and soon fell asleep. I believe it is best to leave her alone when she nods off on the floor while meditating, since we have a big, thick mat that we spread out.

We tried a 'half-soak' (half-bath) in the evening because that's what she wanted. After nearly half of the tub was filled with warm water, Young-hee got in. She told me to make it colder so I drew additional cold water. Her body, however, did not react well. Half-baths require more time than Young-hee is able to devote to them, because her body cannot endure more than a few minutes. She got out of the tub before the water temperature had even stabilized.

Thus, whether she can have a half-bath depends on how her body is feeling. Yesterday's bathing experience differed starkly from last Monday's, resulting in an unanticipated surprise. On Monday night she claimed that when she submerged in water up to her neck, her muscles could relax; and shortly after the bath, she fell sound asleep. But the contrast between yesterday and today was as pronounced as night and day.

She had trouble falling asleep tonight. Once Young-hee had taken her medication at around 10:00 pm, our daughter stopped by the room with her puppy named Hae-ri, and the two of them engaged in some light conversation and laughter. Young-hee tried to fall asleep after settling into bed at 11:30 pm, but was unsuccessful.

Young-hee's arms and legs never stopped moving. It was saddening to see. After getting all ready for bed, sleep would not come because her neck muscles were active, and her neck and shoulders were tensed up.

I continued to sing "The Lord's Prayer" in a hushed voice. She suggested she ought to take one more Alpram. After giving herself another dose of medication, I whispered to Young-hee as she lay back down:

"You've had a nice life for more than 70 years. You have a husband, you have a son and daughter who are both high achievers, and you've accomplished a lot. You're just going through a rough patch right now. Everything will vanish eventually and become a thing of the past. Never feel that you're alone."

"I'm going to sleep now."

As Young-hee lay there, she gave me a hug and a kiss. I went outside. While writing today's journal entry, I briefly went back into the bedroom and discovered that she was sound asleep and snoring. It made me feel at peace. (7. 31.)

You Have No Idea How Difficult It Is

*"But when you're lying down all day, and people around
you accept it as normal, there's no way out from it."*

Stop It, I'm Tired!

WAS SO TIRED THAT I woke up at 9:30 am. With our daughter's
help, Young-hee had already eaten breakfast. Since she began
having trouble falling asleep at night, Young-hee has exhibited less
will to live, less strength, and less vitality. Not very encouraging . . .

Her face no longer looks full. She does not go outside anymore
and only gives her face a cursory wash. How could she have any
energy? I am desperate to see Young-hee learn how to empty her
mind, let go of her stress, and let go of her obsessions. It hurts to
watch her lose her vibrancy.

I had to go out today. My research assistants needed me at
a meeting. I spoke with Young-hee before leaving for the office.

"Let's go to work together on Tuesdays starting next week.
Let's spend some time at the research center meeting the staff.
We can look over reports, have a few short chats, and then come
back home. You can lie down on the couch in the seminar room
and still talk to people."

I know it is not healthy for her to return to work right away.
But for Young-hee to completely let everything go and struggle
with her movement disorder all day long alone at home—I don't
think it is right.

I wrote Prof. Park of Dongguk University Ilsan Hospital an email as soon as I arrived at the office. I briefed her on the current situation and told her about our meeting with Prof. Jeon. I also informed her about my wife's sleeping issues, especially at night.

Unexpectedly, Prof. Park called me back. She said that she had reviewed the recent treatment history after getting my letter. First off, in regards to the issue with Young-hee's sleep, she advised her to take two Alpram pills three times per day and promised to write a prescription for more. She continued by stating that if it was difficult for the patient to arrive before noon on August 2, a family member might do so in her place. She would only be on duty in the morning. I explained that my wife would have her BATAE breathing exercise session tomorrow at 10:00 am, thus I would only be able to go in the afternoon. In that case, Prof. Park advised me to come to the office in the afternoon and that she would have the prescription ready for me. I thanked the doctor.

I finished work at around 4:00 pm. Young-hee was lying down in the room. "You must have been busy today", she said as she welcomed me. Repeating what I had said in the morning, I mentioned that everyone was looking forward to seeing her in the lab at least once a week. I intended to record the visit on video and thought we could have a relaxed conversation about it, but when I suggested it to Young-hee, she did not seem interested. She was having a lot of issues with her body.

At that point, the dialogue ought to have ended. But I persisted.

"We visited Seoul National University Hospital last Monday, where you were able to last for more than three hours without lying down."

It might have sounded a bit like a criticism.

"At the time, I was in a position where I didn't have a choice."

"Wouldn't it be possible to do it again for roughly an hour, lying down as needed, since you did it for more than three hours then?"

"You don't seem to understand how difficult my situation is."

In fact, I was attempting to comprehend her emotions, but how could I? How could I understand how it feels to have a neck so stiff, so sore, and to have one's shoulder and neck move involuntarily? I would ask her if there was any discomfort or aching along with the movement. Young-hee answered that it was not painful. The sensation was more akin to "annoying, heavy, oppressive".

"I'm sure it's incredibly difficult for you . . . It hurts a lot when I'm holding your hand gently, when your muscles start to shake wildly and you're struggling, you grab my hand. When it happens, I feel completely helpless and I know you can't help it or do anything about it. But when you're lying down all day, and people around you accept it as normal, there's no way out from it."

Then Young-hee spat,

"Stop it! I'm tired!"

I quickly came to the realization that I had gone too far. I said I was sorry and backed off.

"I'm sorry! I'm really sorry . . . "

As usual, I took hold of Young-hee's hand as she lay motionless and pulled it forward, then released it. She then performed breathing exercises as I lightly jiggled her hand to relax it, and so on, repeating the cycle numerous times. It wasn't a smooth process. Her body appeared to be struggling.

After dinner, I assisted Young-hee with her arm and leg exercises and started clearing space in the study for the massage bed that will arrive tomorrow. (8. 1.)

Setting Up My Wife's "Sleeping Gym"

YOUNG-HEE WAS SCHEDULED TO BE at BATAE at 10:00 am, but its exercise room was moved yesterday and it wasn't ready yet. Her appointment was rescheduled for 4:00 pm.

I visited Prof. Park of Dongguk University Ilsan Hospital in the morning. She questioned me about the quality of Young-hee's sleep last night. I reported that after taking two Alprams, she had dozed off after a little more than an hour. She then asked how things were in the morning, and I replied that she had to strain while using the toilet, and that when I left the house, her chin and shoulders were active. Prof. Park's new prescription was as follows:

> "Increase the dosage of Alpram to 0.5 milligrams
> and take it with Rivotril and Lexapro after breakfast.
> Increase the dosage of the Alpram to 0.5 milligrams and
> take it right after lunch and before bed. She can take a
> Rivotril tablet if she is having problems falling asleep.

Rivotril takes time to work but lasts a long time, while Alpram works immediately and wears off quickly.

Even very heavy pressure applied during a neck massage or acupressure isn't necessarily a concern if there are no indications of pain in the muscles. Pain may not be felt if the muscles are bundled together too tightly or if there are frequent muscle tremors across the shoulders and neck.

The best outcomes for recovery are obtained when the patient bravely moves past her ailment and her focus is redirected, rather than dwelling on her feelings moment by moment. To forget the symptoms, she should take active interest in other things."

Young-hee said her BATAE session went really well. However, she claimed she was having difficulties as usual when she got home. Her shoulders and chin were quaking, especially when she ate dinner. Drinking water posed another problem.

Her arms and body moved from side to side constantly when she lay down, seemingly a result of the neck muscle activity. That is normal. She is unable to move her arms or legs much while sitting, which places further strain and discomfort on her body.

On the other hand, standing and walking gently, moving her shoulders, and slightly lifting her heels, is certain to be more comfortable than sitting down because it involves moving her arms and legs. By the same token, rather than sitting straight up in a chair, it is surely better for her to sit up in bed with her back leaning against the headboard, letting her arms shake and her legs move back and forth.

Seeing Young-hee's limbs swaying involuntarily as she fell asleep was heartbreaking. I wasn't able to do much for her. As I lay by her waiting for the swaying to stop, feeling the warmth of our arms, I moved my arm in sync with whichever way Young-hee's arm was moving. It took an entire hour. When I noticed that Young-hee was feeling more at ease, I said "good night" and got out of bed. As I watched her nod off, I felt at peace, too. I shut off the A/C and set about doing my own work.

But, when Young-hee fell asleep, it meant leaving me behind. Although it was cozy for her, we grew apart, we became strangers. We could not experience the same emotions. On the other hand, we could see and feel one another when we moved around on the bed. It was difficult emotionally, but the moving around was like a form of exercise, a rite of passage in preparation for sleep. 'Ah, Young-hee is exercising to help her sleep.' Thinking of it that way lessened the terribleness of the situation.

But then Young-hee said,

"You, move away from me."

I read this to mean 'stay away' because my skin felt hot against hers.

"You need to get out of the bed and give me space to move."

"Oh, yes, it's your exercise time! I'll get out of the way so you can move around however you like."

I went to the study and spent some time online. Before long, I noticed that an hour had passed since she had taken her medication. Young-hee's body was still moving left and right when I entered the bedroom.

"Before you know it, you'll be asleep."

I spent a short while lying on the floor, my legs up and feet resting on the bed.

Young-hee's body eventually calmed down. I returned to the study after turning off the A/C and the fan. (8. 2.)

CHAPTER 4

· · ·

How We Can Be Different

There Are Good Days and Bad Days

"It's tough, but whenever you go out, you always manage yourself quite well: you don't lie down, you sit or you walk slowly, and you keep up with the schedule. I wonder— what if you lived a more regular life?"

Variations of Expectation and Disappointment

TODAY WE SEE THE RESULTS of the new experiment. She took two pills before going to bed last night. Her arms and legs swayed for more than an hour before going to sleep, but it was still better than before. We had always been anxious about taking a second pill when the first one didn't work, but now a double dose is permitted.

I was the first one to wake up this morning. Young-hee was still fast asleep. I rolled over and slept some more.

Around 9:30 am, when I woke up again, Young-hee was up on her feet, walking around slowly and chewing some *Gongjindan* herbal medicine. We said "good morning". Her muscles are typically not very active in the mornings, but today she felt better than usual. "My neck isn't acting up." It was nice to hear.

After lunch, Young-hee dozed off and did not wake up again until almost 7:00 pm. She had slept for most of the day, which helped to relieve her stiff neck and heavy shoulders.

Young-hee was fully at ease while she watched TV after dinner. She did not fully lie down; she lay at an angle. She appeared to be focusing her attention on the screen rather than on the discomfort in her neck.

We tried the bath again. I wanted to overcome the horror we had been through before. I made the water lukewarm so Young-hee could easily enter the tub. For the first time, we also used a device that was incorporated into the tub. It massages the body with water. It was noisy, but that didn't bother us. I shampooed her hair without Young-hee having to use her hands. A triumph! We then proceeded to the bedroom, where I laid her down, dressed her, and dried her hair. There were no problems.

We watched TV some more, and at about 11:20 pm, before bedtime, she took her last two pills for the day. I anticipated she would nod off in little over an hour. In the past, once she took her medication, I switched off the fluorescent light and the TV and we would try to get to sleep, and it was not easy. Her body would move uncontrollably for an hour or more. But tonight I sat on the bed next to her and we watched a movie.

Young-hee's movements began to slow down after an hour or so. After getting everything in order, I gave Young-hee a good night kiss. Afterwards I had a massage, sitting in the massage chair. The day went very differently compared to yesterday. I wonder how it will be tomorrow. (8. 3.)

Why Are You So Good?

MY HOPES WERE DASHED. TODAY was not at all like yesterday. Young-hee woke up rather early. She looked every bit the patient after the many hours of sleep she got after taking her medication. She was lethargic and walked around very slowly. By 8:40 am, we finished our breakfast. I saw that her neck was quaking as she ate. On mornings when she was in a pleasant mood, she went back and forth between the bedroom and the study. Today, though, she went back and lay down right after breakfast.

She took her medication at 9:20 am and struggled until eventually dozing off at 10:40 am. She woke up again at 12:40 pm, an hour earlier than yesterday. Normally, after she sleeps, her body feels more relaxed, but today, that was not the case.

"I took my medicine but no let-up . . . "

Young-hee is very sensitive about her physical condition. Even drinking water was more difficult today than yesterday.

Our daughter helped with lunch but Young-hee's body was noticeably shaking. The contour of her mouth was also unnatural when she took food. Nonetheless, she completed her dinner successfully.

While I lay next to her, Young-hee asked me to help her move her right arm so she could exercise it. She took hold of my left arm with her right hand and began forcing my arm to move with hers. The arm had strength. Its muscles shook with a terrifying energy. Things were now more serious than a quaking jaw. I tried to release any resistance in my body and mind, and let Young-hee's arm and hand guide mine wherever they saw fit.

Despite the difficulty, Young-hee occasionally stood up, drank some water, and moved slowly around the room, exercising her arms and shoulders. But she could not go on like this for very long.

"I know it's incredibly hard right now, but I'm scared that you will lose your strength. Your leg muscles will weaken, and then one day you'll fall and it will be serious. Moving around and losing weight are good for your health, but you shouldn't let your muscles deteriorate. It will lead to other issues.

It's tough, but whenever you go out, you always manage yourself quite well: you don't lie down, you sit or you walk slowly, and you keep up with the schedule. I wonder—what if you lived a more regular life? Naturally, you shouldn't overdo it, but you shouldn't spend your entire day in bed, either. Even a little movement can reduce your stress and make you tired, and can help you sleep better."

To that end, I suggested that we go to the National Library, which is close to our apartment building.

"It must be hot out . . . "

"Mr. Kim will drive us."

At such times, Young-hee exhibited a tendency toward timidity and dread.

To make it to Seoul National University Hospital by 9:00 tomorrow, we had to go to bed early. I questioned Young-hee as she lay next to me about something I had been meaning to ask her.

"Do you like it when I'm lying down next to you, us holding each other, or do you prefer letting your hands and feet sway on the bed alone? Which do you feel more at ease with?"

"When you're by me, I feel like I'm relying on you. I like that."

"Then I'll be by you around the clock."

"You have a job."

"No, I've worked too much lately. I need to be with you now."

Young-hee said thank you. She said she was about to cry.

"It's what a husband should do."

"Why are you so good to me?"

"Good? I'm simply doing my duty. The subject of pain is one that religions take very seriously. 'Why is there so much pain in human life, and what does it all mean?' That's the foundation of religion. Suffering isn't something to be feared or avoided. It teaches the forgiveness of sins, the cleansing of the body and mind, and a positive attitude that is open to receiving grace and seeking salvation. I think you share my sentiments. When you said that you 'must have sinned a lot', for example."

I continued,

"You haven't wronged me at all. You are, after all, my blessing. We've gone through a lot academically and socially together, and you gave birth to our son and daughter."

"No, I've wronged you in so many ways."

"What ways are you referring to? You're innocent of any wrongdoing."

"I get ahead of myself and make you follow . . . "

Young-hee appeared to be thinking a lot as she struggled to keep control of her worn-out body.

It was close to 11:00 pm.

"You'll soon drop off to sleep. Stay relaxed and calm. I'll stay by you."

"Right, you're Shim Young-hee's husband!"

"Yes. Yes. Well, then. Good night." (8. 4.)

There Are Faint But Small Noticeable Changes Now!

"The unexpected had happened. She had tested out the tool on her own while I was out exercising. Concealing a smile, I shifted my body to demonstrate the correct form. We did the exercise together."

My Wife Shows a Willingness to Take Care of Herself

I WENT TO BED LAST NIGHT—ACTUALLY, at 3:30 this morning—and woke up at 7:00 am. Young-hee had an appointment at Seoul National University Hospital today. She had to be at the hospital by 9:00 am for the autoimmune test, which required fluid to be drawn from her spinal cord. She was informed that following the treatment, she would need to be in a lying position for four hours. It looked like it might be a grueling day.

When Young-hee is compelled to act, she handles it admirably—outside more than at home. Sometimes she continues to do well after the pressure is off. I watched Young-hee, our daughter, and our daughter-in-law leave for the hospital, wondering how the day would conclude. For the first time in a long while, I also went to work.

At 3:00 pm, I visited the hospital. The spinal fluid extraction, fortunately, went smoothly. At 3:50, she was told she could leave. Young-hee was in good spirits, as I had hoped. She had handled herself well and persevered through the day. After many hours of fasting, she was finally permitted to sip some water when she was discharged from the hospital. She had skipped lunch, so she was hungry.

It was about 5:00 pm when she finished eating, and she was in rather good condition when she lay down to rest. Young-hee was not in bad shape at all. I moved her right hand around and raised her arms above her head. For a few moments, she stood up and walked gently about the room, doing her neck and arm exercises.

By 11:00 pm, Young-hee's body appeared to quiet down. I switched off the TV.

"Why did you turn the TV off?"

"I figured it was time for bed."

"No, I want to keep watching."

"Oh. I'll turn it back on then, of course."

Welcome words. I wanted Young-hee to watch the TV and go to sleep without thinking or worrying. It was much better than struggling to fall asleep. I wondered about the day that lay ahead. (8. 5.)

Young-hee's condition was not bad this morning. Some new herbal medicines arrived by post. She took some of them before her shower. We had to go to Seoul National University Hospital again this morning since the medical staff forgot to draw Young-hee's blood before her release yesterday.

Prof. Jeon's assistant was waiting for us when we got there. Young-hee had her blood drawn and then came straight home. I made a brief stop to see my brother, who is a patient at the same hospital, before heading to Ewha Womans University to see a friend and give her a copy of my book.

The family was having dinner when I got home. Young-hee said that after lunch, while she was meditating, she had grown tired and had a 3-hour nap without taking her afternoon medication. It appears that the effects from the morning dose took hold.

I enjoyed dinner. Yet, it was not all lightness. Since she was moving slowly, swinging her arms, rotating her shoulders, and slightly lifting and lowering her heels, Young-hee's neck felt less stiff and her arms did not seem as heavy. But, she felt vaguely ill at ease. She said that she could not take a bath. She occasionally asked for help in rotating her arm.

The much-awaited massage bed arrived. After setting it up, it stood a lot taller than I expected. (8. 6.)

Just the Thing: Active Muscle Strengthening

I HAD LUNCH, SPENT SOME TIME alone outside, and then came right home. Young-hee was awake, standing in the bedroom, sipping some water.

"You're back in a hurry. I slept a little."

"I did what I had to do and came home. Did you get a lot of rest?"

"About two hours."

It was good news. She had just woken up, so her condition did not look bad. She asked me to help her manipulate her arms. As I helped her with this and that task, I reminded her:

"You have a new exercise tool, you know. I hope you learn how to use it. I can help you, but if you use it consistently as recommended, in keeping with your physical state, it can help you. Ultimately, you'll have to decide for yourself, based on how your body feels."

But Young-hee didn't seem to be planning to put the TRX she had borrowed from BATAE to the test. She was watching TV, curled up on the couch, her limbs trembling. Of course, it was nice to see her watching TV. But I had just set up the new tool, so inwardly, I expected her to get up and use it.

"Well, should we give it a shot? Look it over. How does it seem to you?"

I lay on the bed with a large cushion behind me, and watched TV with her. My body was worn out. I was fatigued from not getting enough sleep, from my own inability to sleep soundly, and from the failure of my plans.

"Now, let's get moving and go for a walk instead of lying around here."

Just as I was about to leave, Young-hee stopped me.

"When are we going to try the thing you installed? You said I couldn't do it alone, didn't you?"

"I can't stand by all the time! Let's get started on it together right now if you want to."

"No, not right this minute."

The weather was scorching. I strolled alongside Banpocheon Stream, stretched my body out at a tiny rest area, and en route home proceeded to the playground to do some laps there. As I did, a thought came to me.

"Today marks a fresh start. A stiff neck and heavy shoulders are a burden, but the condition isn't lethal. It's one that needs to be overcome. Young-hee must navigate the way on her own, using her body's natural breathing and movement patterns. Nobody can instill that will and drive in her. We can try to help, but if she doesn't take the necessary steps by herself, we should treat her firmly and dispassionately. The path ahead will be hard for her if she makes no effort at all. True, she will have to struggle at first if she decides to exercise her own willpower and learn and practice, but doing just that will help her, by tiring her out and making it easier for her to sleep. If she relaxes her muscles while she sleeps, and exercises slowly and consistently to control her muscles while she's awake, this, together with the effects of her medications, will ultimately help her restore her body to normal."

I assisted Young-hee with neck and arm stretches after dinner and gently paced with her around the bedroom.

As we spent time watching TV, 10:00 pm rolled around. She took one pill.

"Let's do some light exercises with the new tool after you take your medication. The focus should be on breathing and exhaling in order to relax, not on motion or using your strength. It's not hot since we're doing it indoors, and if you get tired, you can just lie down on the bed. Let's conduct it as an experiment."

"OK, but I've already tried it."

The unexpected had happened. She had tested out the tool on her own while I was out exercising. Concealing a smile, I shifted my body to demonstrate the correct form. We did the exercise together.

"Ow, it's killing me."

Young-hee was unable to continue for very long. She immediately sank back onto the bed.

I was happy. My wish had been granted. (8. 7.)

Change Me, Lord, Not the Circumstance

"She could barely feel any strength in her left arm, a dull sensation in her fingers, and difficulty moving her left shoulder due to what she believes to be congestion between her shoulder blades."

Hoping for a Miracle Is Greedy

WE DID NOT PLAN TO go anywhere today. We both woke up later than usual for a weekday. This morning, Young-hee's condition was pretty good, so we both had a bath. Young-hee said it felt good. After shampooing and drying her hair, I helped her get dressed while she lay on the bed. I also applied lotion to her hands.

But now she announced that her left arm was giving her trouble. She claimed that her left shoulder blade was in pain. I speculated that it might be related to the way she slept, or to the exercise she did yesterday. Young-hee's neck frequently stiffens up because of her constant anxiety about physical changes in her body. I pointed out to her that I am also struggling with a tight neck and heavy shoulders. I tried to reassure her by reminding her that rehabilitation is often an up-and-down process.

We had breakfast after 10:00 am. Young-hee decided that she would take her morning dose so that her body would not feel 'off', and took a 0.25 mg tablet along with her other medication. She wanted to sleep a little better during her naptime.

She lay down again after lunch, complaining again that something felt off with her left arm. Then, around 2:40 pm, she tried to sleep. She quickly dozed off when I repositioned her right arm and hand, which were causing her discomfort. I also stretched out her left arm gently. After two hours, Young-hee woke up.

"Where are you going?"

"I have to go to church . . ."

"OK, have a nice time."

It pained me to sing "The Lord's Prayer" alone at Mass because we had always sung it together, holding hands. Young-hee had trouble staying still, particularly while standing. Her body swayed back and forth. Others held their bodies upright while praying. Only Young-hee swayed. Yes, I thought. Why hadn't I seen that this was a precursor to her condition now? She had sent clear signals, and my failure to notice them hurt me deeply. The priest announced that he would shorten the homily since it was such a hot day. He explained how to pray.

"We will inevitably run into difficult circumstances as we navigate through life, and pleading with God to alter our circumstance is tantamount to seeking a miracle. To get through difficult situations, the essential posture of prayer is to ask God to keep changing me, rather than asking Him to end the circumstance with a snap of the fingers. The essence of prayer, and its power, lies in changing oneself in accordance with God's will."

The homily's message rang true to my heart. It is far too easy for us to criticize, to feel resentment toward others, when we feel irritated or offended. When we turn it around and motivate ourselves to change, our hearts grow lighter. When we pray for ourselves to change, our anger at other people disappears. I needed to be in that mindset when caring for Young-hee.

Young-hee took her medication in the evening, dozed off, and then woke up about two hours later to use the bathroom. She made an attempt to fall back asleep, but failed. I gently repositioned Young-hee's right arm and hand. When she noticed that I was still awake, it must have concerned her, because she told me, "Alright, you sleep now".

"No, no problem. After you go to sleep, I have to turn off the air conditioner, anyway. Don't fret about it."

I carried out the same motions while lying next to Young-hee. She quickly dropped off again. I thought to myself. "Alright, you sleep now" is Young-hee's manner of speaking. She constantly views herself as a subject who "instructs" others. It is an old habit. She is always in a place where she is either supervising other people or doing something herself. She makes the decisions. Receptive speech—phrases like "Thank you", and questions like "Aren't you tired?"—while not wholly alien to her, is not 'typical Young-hee' behavior, plain and simple.

Letting go of everything, following the other person rather than being the subject who stands over them, letting the other person do what they want rather than telling them what to do—these seem to be crucial skills for Young-hee to acquire. *Let everything go. Empty yourself.* The words are simple to say. But, taking action is challenging. These are undoubtedly formidable tasks for me, as well. (8. 11.)

The Night Comes When She Can Sleep Alone

YOUNG-HEE AND OUR DAUGHTER WENT to BATAE together. They returned the TRX tool that Young-hee had borrowed, and returned home around 12:20 pm.

"How was it? Was it good today?"

"Ah, much better. We did a lot of breathing exercises. Are you going to work? Contact Mr. Kim."

She meant that she was doing fine and she wanted me to go to the lab. I texted the department after lunch and let them know I would be at work at 1:00 pm.

I arrived home around 6:30. Young-hee's face was beaming. In our bedroom, our grandchildren were using their tablets to play games. Young-hee was on her feet, holding on to a pole, and slowly rocking back and forth. Our son's family went back home after dinner.

We watched an entertainment program together. Young-hee did not ask for help with her hand this evening, she was much more at ease with a lot more wherewithal to concentrate on the TV. Her legs and arms were comparatively calm. Young-hee used the TRX apparatus to exercise. As I leaned back, she leaned backwards against my chest and let out a tension-relaxing breath. She repeated this several times.

At 9:40 pm, she took one pill. As she lay in bed watching TV, she grew sleepy. I sat down next to her so I could gently move her arms and hands. Her legs also calmed down. I switched everything off and covered her with a blanket.

"Why did you turn off the TV?"

119

I was mistaken in thinking that she was asleep. She mentioned that her legs felt funny, so I turned the A/C and TV back on and kept an eye on her legs. Periodically, her right leg trembled, a lot like her troublesome right arm. I placed a rolling pin made of cypress wood under her calves and let her to roll on it to massage her leg, as she had done before.

Her limbs typically moved from side to side as she fell asleep at night, but this particular evening they were very still. My mind at peace, I went out to the study. By 11:30 pm, when I returned to the bedroom, Young-hee was fast asleep. (8. 12.)

Why I Need to Be Stronger

I T WAS A DAY FILLED with ups and downs. It was a happy time of the day when Young-hee and I went for a quick stroll around the apartment complex and garden, and then over to the Cloud Cafe to have a cup of tea.

At nighttime, though, the worst came to the worst. Young-hee experienced respiratory issues and it threw her into a panic. She was in misery, and crying.

There are two things I must remember.

First, on days when Young-hee and I are at home together, all of my thoughts must be on her. She put a lot of strain on her throat this morning. When she woke up from sleep at 5:30 pm feeling out of sorts, she got up and yelled for our daughter from the bedroom doorway. This made the muscles in Young-hee's neck grow extremely tense. It could have been avoided if I had been by her side.

Second, in light of her psychological state, we must devise a method for Young-hee to contact us when she needs us. I will come up with a plan so that when Young-hee presses a button, our daughter's room receives a signal. (8. 15.)

I slept in late this morning because I was so tired. In light of yesterday's experience, I reasoned that it would be best for Young-hee to avoid taking a shower that required a lot of touching and scrubbing. Young-hee wanted to take a shower, but she had to be at BATAE by 11:00 am.

Young-hee came back with our daughter at 12:30. She said that despite her best efforts to relax her tense muscles, she had not had much success—a lingering effect from yesterday's ordeal. Young-hee spent much of the day in bed, her neck muscles still throbbing aggressively.

Young-hee's right arm has been a main source of trouble. Her right arm experiences severe pain resulting from the violent activity of the muscles on the right side of her neck. She grabs my hand and jerks it back and forth vigorously alongside her own. Her left arm, though, has had fewer difficulties. But today Young-hee noted that her left arm was giving her strange sensations, just like two days ago. She could barely feel any strength in her left arm, a dull sensation in her fingers, and difficulty moving her left shoulder due to what she believes to be congestion between her shoulder blades. She added that it was difficult for her to move her arm back and forth. Her posture is obviously skewed and unnatural. Cantankerous spirits seemed to be wreaking havoc on Young-hee's muscles.

Today she took one 0.5 mg Alpram tablet at around 8:40 pm, deciding to take her medication as soon as possible. She then took one pill at lunch and another at dinner. Around an hour to an hour-and-a-half later, she started feeling drowsy.

We watched her favorite channel to distract her from her pain. Just being able to do this was a significant improvement from before.

I went to Banpo Stadium sometime after 11:00 pm to relieve my physical fatigue and discomfort. It was breezy and cool. I took a 40-minute stroll. I had not been outside for a while and was thinking about a lot of things as I walked:

"My body may sometimes feel out of sorts, but I certainly shouldn't let the sick Young-hee see me looking run-down if I don't have to. I occasionally catch Young-hee observing my facial expressions and thinking to herself. If I appear to struggle, this will cause Young-hee difficulty, too. She needs to be free to direct me in what I need to do and how I should behave. In order to prevent the psychological weight that my suffering—caused by Young-hee—places on her, I must always embrace her fully with my actions and my heart."

This led me to recall the homily from the previous week. It is better to pray, "God, change me", than to pray for this challenging circumstance to change. (8. 16.)

The 'Here and Now' Is Our Paradise

"Young-hee extended her right hand in search of something to hold on to and pull on. My hand was just the thing. The moment I saw her hand, I recognized that Young-hee was calling out to me."

The Breeze, That Refreshing Taste of Living

WENT FOR A WALK ALONE along Banpocheon Trail in the morning and returned home just after 1:00 pm. I found our daughter preparing lunch. Today, lunch was served later than usual. As she ate, Young-hee's condition did not appear to be particularly bad, but it was not good either.

She was taking food in her mouth from our daughter while seated on a chair, her hands behind her back, clenching the edge of the seat. She seemed more at ease with her hands there than under or on top of the table. After the meal, I asked Young-hee about it. She explained that sitting in that position was the most comfortable for her, but she couldn't maintain it for very long.

"But didn't you sit like that throughout your meal?"

I questioned her, seeing that sitting upright in the chair was an important task for her.

"It wasn't easy. I was barely hanging on!"

"Yes . . ."

I let the matter drop. A few times, while we watched television, she signaled to me to tug on her arm. She seemed to be having a hard time of it. Young-hee sighed with exhaustion.

"Do I need to take Alpram today?"

"Of course, you should if you're tired."

I gathered that she wanted to take her medication and just go to bed.

In the evening, the weather was cool, so we decided to spend some time outside. A refreshing wind was blowing when we exited the first floor entrance and stepped outside. Young-hee welcomed it. She took in a long, deep breath and rotated her arms to the left and right, then up and down.

"Cool air . . . it tastes like living", she said.

When muscles are working hard, they typically get warm and produce perspiration, and Young-hee found the crispness of the outdoor air a great joy. But that did not last for long. Initially, we were able to complete one lap of the elliptical garden in front of our building.

Young-hee and I do a stress-relieving exercise where we hold hands. We did it twice. I use my strength in the exercise, and Young-hee releases hers. Young-hee suddenly bent down and then raised her arms behind her. I was happy that she was taking the initiative to do that.

"Good! Outstanding!"

But, at that point, Young-hee's countenance changed, signifying she was having a problem—a little breathing difficulty. The exercise, involving the use of strength, caused her neck muscles to jerk and throb in reaction. Young-hee immediately acknowledged her condition and asked that we go back. We quickly did some stretches by the neighboring playground before heading home.

Young-hee took her medication at 9:10 pm. I used the TRX for a while to relax my hands, feet, shoulders, and back, while observing Young-hee as she watched TV on the floor next to the bed. Young-hee occasionally laughed when she saw something funny. It was encouraging to see that she was moving past her health issues and showing interest in other things. I figured we might even go to work together at some point.

Saddest of all, Young-hee's right arm continued to sway in the air while she watched TV. Young-hee extended her right hand in search of something to hold on to and pull on. My hand was just the thing. The moment I saw her hand, I recognized that Young-hee was calling out to me.

I hope that Young-hee picks up using the TRX fast and gives her right arm the exercise it needs. But it will probably take some time.

I wanted to go for a walk, so I went to Banpo Stadium. Today, there was almost no one there, just a full moon visible in the sky. I naturally had a talk with God in my head and heart.

I believe that when Young-hee recovers, she will live a more responsible life. Might there be a new beginning in the offing? Nowadays, I talk about transformation, and have entertained the possibility that one might occur in my life. (8. 17.)

A Time So Precious in Our Life

YOUNG-HEE WAS THE FIRST TO awaken. Our daughter attended to breakfast. Watching Young-hee eat breakfast was pleasant. She enjoyed her meal and had some watermelon for dessert. Although it was a cool day, I switched on the A/Cs in the dining room and bedroom for Young-hee's health.

The day got off to a great start, but soon another challenge arose. Before breakfast, Young-hee made an attempt to have a bowel movement, but to no avail. After breakfast, she went to the bathroom again and spent quite a bit of energy, hoping to pass some stool. This time she succeeded, but all the energy she spent could have led to a serious problem.

I attempted to brush her teeth for her, but she refused and did it on her own. Young-hee, mouth open wide, put a lot of energy into the task. Soon, she was gasping for air.

Young-hee needed help to breathe. I quickly led her out of the bathroom and laid her down, but it was not enough.

Young-hee eventually broke out in tears. All I could do was give her a hug.

She sobbed bitterly for a long while. I stood at her side, dabbing her tears away.

In time, she began to calm down, but her right arm and hand continued to flail out of control.

"OK, then, should we switch on the TV?"

Young-hee nodded and smiled. She felt better.

"You're struggling because of me, aren't you?"

"Because of the unusual positions, I ... my back feels strange sometimes."

I lay down close to Young-hee. She grabbed my hand and squeezed it.

"You should exercise. Come exercise ... "

In truth, the weather was cool, and I had been thinking about taking a walk outdoors since morning.

"How am I supposed to go out with you, in this state?"

"Then use the TRX."

"Good idea!"

I began warming up with the TRX in the hallway by the bedroom door. I pulled, leaned, hung, sat, and stood, while Young-hee watched TV ... We occasionally chuckled when our eyes met.

I discovered then that the space we shared—the bedroom, the study, and the hallway between—was in fact our paradise. We have a living room and a dining room in our rather sizable apartment. One of the small rooms is a kind of reading area crammed full of books.

Our daughter uses another room, and across from it, a separate room for her family, Meon-ji, Hae-ri, and Yul-li. The living room and the rooms we use are separated by a door that opens to a hallway that connects our bedroom on the right to the study on the left. I hang the TRX on the study door, then I close the door to secure it in place. I exercise while facing the bedroom, sometimes watching Young-hee as I do my routine. I can do a variety of workouts here.

When was the last time we spent so much time together, shared our thoughts and feelings, were so close? Even when we were together, we were frequently so busy that we hardly ever had the chance to share moments that unified our hearts and minds. But now we spend the entire day cooperating as a team. It is how we approach each passing moment.

This is our paradise, I thought. When our two hearts are united, our worries and fears vanish; we do not fear death; and it seems like happiness can be ours, despite any obstacle that may stand in our way. Suddenly, the suffering seems like a blessing!

In the evening, while watching TV, Young-hee occasionally motioned to me to tug on her hand. I spend virtually the entire day by her side because she needs me. She often motions anxiously to me with her hand when things get tough. Young-hee is always trying to grab my hand. When we hold hands, her psychological condition seems to improve.

"Without you, I feel anxious."

"Don't worry. I'll stand by you always."

"You need to go to your job. You need to visit China as well."

"I don't have to go to work; and as for China, I'll say I won't go."

I will do anything for Young-hee, but dependence like this is not always a good thing. I made the TRX strap longer so that it reaches the bed. That way, she can lie down and grasp something when I am not here to hold her hand. I advised Young-hee to lie down and test it. She "gave it a try" several times, but found it unwieldy.

Since she had a late dinner, she took her medication around 9:30 pm. I felt she was going to fall asleep, but that didn't happen. She then took a Rivotril, her second dose, at midnight.

"I can't sleep tonight."

After the second Rivotril, there was nothing else she could take to fall asleep. I silently left the bedroom to go to the study. When I came back, a dozing Young-hee was lying on the floor, on the mat at the foot of the bed, her right foot propped up, resting on the mattress.

Young-hee must have had a terrible day. Today, though, I realized that "this is my paradise". (8. 18.)

CHAPTER 5

. . .

I'm By Your Side

Music To My Ears: "Shall We Go Outside?"

"After dinner, the weather outside was not terribly hot.
When I suggested going out, Young-hee willingly
followed. Today, though, she took a pill beforehand."

Our Arms and Hearts Together as One

Young-hee said that she felt better after her BATAE session. Good news.

A short while afterwards, our son dropped by. Big-hearted and kind-natured, he is particularly sensitive to his mother's health problems. He exhibited considerable skepticism about the therapy process and often questioned whether the prescribed drugs were actually having a healing effect. I voiced my thoughts:

"We're moving toward the healing phase now. There's no one size fits all answer when it comes to how a prescription will affect a patient. Every patient is different, just as every healing procedure is different . . . Let's be patient, take our time, and have faith in the medical professionals. If we mistrust the doctor because we don't see immediate results, it could be a formula for disaster.

Now is the time to investigate her problems from a variety of angles as we look for ways to make your mother's daily life better. There have been noticeable improvements. It's simpler now to anticipate how to respond when she feels intense physical discomfort, panic episodes, and, of course, the difficult process of falling asleep at night. Finding a means for your mother to sit and pass the time comfortably is of the utmost importance right now, since lying down all day can lead to a host of other problems.

Her daily life—not rehabilitation—is what matters now. Healing should focus on helping your mother with her everyday tasks, while keeping faith that the doctor's prescriptions and advice will eventually take effect."

My son advised hiring a caregiver, since it wouldn't cost too much. I concurred that it was a reasonable idea, even though I preferred that we handle the situation as a family.

"I want to use it as an opportunity for us to come together, to unite our hearts and minds, to be born again."

When I got back from my afternoon outing, Young-hee was not in the best of shape. She felt a lot of muscle pressure in her right arm. She experiences this pressure constantly, with the exception of when she sleeps and for a short while when she wakes up. Such a sad sight. I wiped the perspiration from her forehead and caressed her face with my two hands.

I suggested that if the A/C was not helping, we should turn it off and let some outside air in. The weather was not as pleasant as yesterday, but not unbearably hot either. Young-hee commented on how nice the crisp air felt. To keep the room at a comfortable temperature, I left the fan on. But then something strange happened.

"Shall we go outside?"

Such welcome words! It was a sign that Young-hee's heart was turning to face the outside world.

"We can go outside even though the weather's not cool."

Together, we went down to the first floor. This time it wasn't as refreshing because there was no cool wind blowing. After we had walked a while, Young-hee said,

"Hold my right arm as we go."

Something struck me at that very moment. To help Young-hee fall asleep at night, I frequently have taken her right arm and hand in mine, and gently move and exercise them. Her right arm gives her the most trouble. It is now stuck by her side and does not move. To help Young-hee walk, I had to somehow move it away from her waist. Walking on her right side, I supported her right wrist with my left hand and helped her raise and lower her right arm with my other hand. But there was a lot of resistance because Young-hee's right arm was practically glued to her side. The arm wanted to go back to where it was.

I had to adapt to the resistance of her muscles. Young-hee found it difficult to fight against the pressure, and I found it extremely so as well.

Dealing with her left arm was less of a problem. Switching sides to stand on her left, I used my right hand to raise and lower her left arm above her head in sync with her steps, which required me to swing my left arm back and forth vigorously.

It felt amazing, according to Young-hee. It worked wonderfully. After all, the idea was simple. Young-hee appeared to feel some relief from the tension in her shoulders as she moved her outstretched right arm up and down effortlessly, letting me do all the work. Her left arm was the same way. She felt her shoulders relax and her steps become lighter as a result. We happened upon this new technique by trial and error. I experienced a fresh hope.

"Can we go two rounds around Banpo Stadium like this?"

Once more, after getting back home, we encountered a number of surprises. We had walked for a very long time compared to what was typical, and it had undoubtedly been exhausting. Young-hee lay down immediately. I tried to move Young-hee's arms, raising, lowering, and tugging at them. Oddly, though, her hands and arms barely registered any of the strain from the ferocious activity in her neck muscles. Her right arm was free from pressure. Her body was worn out and she nodded off easily.

"Your hands and arms are much calmer now. Don't you feel it?"

Young-hee said the same. We retired to bed. I gently held Young-hee's hand and wrist and exercised them. Her hand went still after about two minutes. It took her no time at all to fall asleep. (8. 19.)

Walk, Walk, Walk!

ABOUT 3:00 AM, I WENT to sleep. I had just finished putting on my pajamas when, as I had anticipated, Young-hee awoke to use the bathroom. She then peacefully slipped back into sleep.

About 9:00 am, Young-hee woke up. I had already gotten up and opened the study and bedroom windows to let in fresh air. Young-hee appeared to be in good condition. I considered what I should do moving forward, in light of my observations.

"She should not exert too much force when she has a bowel movement. She should not need to strain to pass her stools if she eats well. She must not strain her head when using a toothbrush to clean her teeth. She should not brush vigorously with her mouth open. This excites the neck muscles and requires energy. When eating, she should not open her mouth too wide. She needs to lower her head a little. Because the muscles in her neck are all interconnected, she should use as little force as possible when she moves, eats, and drinks."

I thought it would be a good idea to apply what we learned yesterday and have one person place the food in Young-hee's mouth while the other extends her right arm out horizontally in front of her and gently moves her left hand up and down. These simple things would make a big difference, I reasoned.

Our daughter saw to Young-hee's food at the table while I held out her right arm horizontally and moved her left hand up and down. Young-hee found it easier to eat that way. As I was holding Young-hee's arm during the meal and attentively feeling the movement in her muscles, I realized that the impact communicated to my hands was noticeably different when she chewed soft foods compared to harder foods. When she ate slowly, with her mouth slightly closed and her head lowered, the intensity in her arm was different from when she ate quickly with her mouth open wide. There seemed to be a lot of things working together.

After dinner, the weather outside was not terribly hot. When I suggested going out, Young-hee willingly followed. Today, though, she took a pill beforehand.

As we were leaving the apartment, our daughter, noticing her mother's poor demeanor and clumsy gait, worriedly questioned whether leaving the house in such a state was a good idea.

But we went out. The breeze was neither cool nor particularly brisk. We set out, walking slowly, keeping Young-hee's right arm level. The initial pressure was so great that Young-hee and I both struggled. But with time, things improved. Her steps became more confident, and her arms relaxed. The situation suddenly looked brighter.

As a result, our second evening stroll was a success. Young-hee must have found it challenging since as soon as we arrived back home, she made a bee-line to our daughter's room near the entranceway and lay down. The A/C was already on and it was pleasant. When I pulled on Young-hee's arm, it was very supple and relaxed.

Although it seemed like Young-hee would fall asleep in a flash, she was unable to do so. I crossed over to the study to get out of her way. After some time, I discovered Young-hee sprawled out on the thick mat in front of the bed.

"Sleeping down here is nicer. It's cooler on the floor."

"Sleep there, then. You'll need to get up to use the bathroom in two hours . . . Since I'll be ready for bed by then, I'll put you back up on the bed." (8. 20.)

What More Can I Do?

"I promise you that you don't have a terminal illness.
It won't kill you. You can get over this ailment with time.
There's no denying that you're getting better."

Turn Off the Radio!

THE ANNUAL MEETING OF THE Korean Society of Social Theory has been going on at the Kangwon National University in Chuncheon since yesterday. I left the apartment before Young-hee awoke because my presentation was today. I gave it in the morning, and then I was asked to lead a panel discussion in the afternoon. When my time was up, I came straight back to Seoul.

I boarded the bus at 5:20 pm and arrived home before 8:00. Our daughter was exercising her mother's right arm, back and forth, up and down, repeatedly. I quickly took over the job.

She took her medication at about 9:00 pm, and then we went for a walk. Young-hee now sees walking favorably. Her positive experiences over the last few days have encouraged her to get outside more and exercise.

It was very cool this evening. Young-hee was in a great mood. I have been getting the knack for soothing her right arm, wrist, and hand. I assisted her in repeating her deep breathing exercises and in moving her arms and legs.

We did a lot of walking. A gentle breeze was blowing that made us feel even better.

When we got home after the day's exertions, Young-hee needed to move around a bit more to relax her body. As she lay on the bed, I assisted her in stretching, bringing her arms up and over her head. I gave her some vitamin C powder that I had dissolved in water. She subsequently asked me about the conference.

"Did you enjoy today's conference? What did the audience think of your presentation? Was there a positive reaction to the Saint-Émilion video? Did you receive a lot of questions?"

She was unusually curious today. The conference had actually been rather dull. There were quite a few participants on the first day, but there were so few people on the second day (today) that things were a little boring. There were some interesting exchanges, though, and while moderating the afternoon session I was provided a lot of food for thought and picked up a lot of knowledge. But I wasn't sure if talking about it right before bedtime was a good idea.

"Not really anything interesting."

After that, I spent some time in the study checking my email. Then, an idea suddenly came to me.

'Young-hee did something she hadn't done in a while—she indicated interest in my attending the conference. What am I doing? I should be telling her all about it!'

I went to Young-hee right away. I pulled her arms over her head and massaged her face with both of my hands.

"Did you want to know about the conference today?"

"Yes!"

"It's time to sleep. I'll fill you in on everything tomorrow."

"No, do it now. I can close my eyes and pay attention."

I began to tell the story of my day from the very beginning, with my bus ride to Chuncheon. I was interrupted by my son and his wife who dropped by for a visit. The four of us chatted about this, that, and the other. During that time, Young-hee was able to somewhat ignore the discomfort caused by her neck tremor.

After they left, Young-hee declared she was tired and was going to fall asleep. It was already past 11:00 pm. We were not sure whether the effects of the previous medication she had taken were still being felt or not. The very power of that suggestion kept Young-hee from dozing off.

"There's no way to tell! Hurry and take your other pill!"

About 11:20 pm, she took her other pill but still could not sleep. I must have looked pretty spent myself, because Young-hee told me to go to sleep before her.

To give her some space and help her feel more at ease, I briefly went to the study. But she yelled out again.

"Honey!"

In fact, my back hurt and I was drained. I lay down by her and took her hand. I cleared my thoughts and let my hand flow in sync with hers. Young-hee was aware of my fatigue. I was grateful for her suggestion that I go to sleep first. She was unable to quiet her mind and was concerned that I was not getting enough sleep. And not only that.

"Turn off the radio."

"Why? Is it bothering you?"

"No, but noise is coming from both it and the TV!"

"You should have spoken up! If it disturbs you, I'll turn it off."

"No, just leave it on."

Young-hee dropped off to sleep before midnight. I lay next to her and watched her quietly, alone with my thoughts, for around thirty minutes.

There had hardly been any noise at all. Sometimes she uses phrases like, "Honey, the noise from the car outside is so loud. Close the door, please!" or "That dripping sound! Tighten the water faucet!". Why, when trying to fall asleep, was she giving instructions? She only needs to stay calm and tune out the noise around her. Faint noises stimulate her nerves, suggesting that Young-hee is expressing some pent-up stress or anxiety residing in her subconscious. Perhaps she is in such a mental state that unwinding is simply something she is unable to do. (8. 23.)

Installing a Tension Relief Station in the Bedroom

YOUNG-HEE WOKE UP AT DAWN. She had a fitful sleep. I was asleep the whole time, unaware of anything. We went for a 30-minute walk after breakfast. She claimed that she was unable to relax because her body was bursting with pent-up energy. Walking was not easy today, either.

I accompanied Young-hee to BATAE. The director graciously answered all of my questions. I had seen that Young-hee's hand had the deformed appearance of a crippled person's as she raised it to press an electrical switch on the wall. When I asked him why, he explained that her neck was putting excessive strain on her shoulders, causing unwanted muscular reactions. He assured us that this will gradually get better as she learns to manage her stress.

I was impressed by the strength-training apparatus installed at the BATAE facility. TRX suspension systems are strung at regular intervals from a large structure connecting the four walls and the ceiling. The systems are pulled in and away from the chest, pushed down and raised up, or stretched crosswise or diagonally. I wanted to install one in our bedroom. I reasoned that if we hung up a few straps and attached handles, Young-hee could place her arms and legs inside the handles to increase her comfort level when lying in bed, rather than letting them hover aimlessly in the air. I examined the construction more closely and asked our driver, Mr. Kim, to purchase some poles and screws so that we might install something like it.

Mr. Kim demonstrated his considerable skill in this regard. He erected six poles and connected them in the space in front of our bed. He then fastened straps to the poles, allowing Young-hee to insert her hands and feet in the handles and control them when they are swaying in the air. That is how our bedroom acquired a structure resembling the exercise facility at BATAE. It was a truly ground-breaking idea. The suspended straps act as a kind of reassuring mechanism for Young-hee when she wants to grab hold of something. Once everything was in place, the bedroom was no longer just a bedroom. It is a "lab", a workshop, that helps Young-hee escape her FMD.

It took a good part of the afternoon to set it up. So after dinner, I brought a towel and water bottle, anticipating that we would take a walk. However, Young-hee still looked ill at ease. As she clung on one of the poles set up in the bedroom, she was not exactly beaming with contentment. She threw a brief tantrum.

"Why are you keeping me waiting like this? Can't you move it along?"

I searched Young-hee's facial expression.

"Lie down and take a nap if you're tired."

Young-hee lay down on the mat by the bed, where it was cooler.

As I pulled on Young-hee's arm, I tried to help her get through the problem she was facing.

"You don't have to go out. Just lie down if you're not in the mood."

Maybe We Need a Caregiver

IN ACTUALITY, YOUNG-HEE HAD BEEN unwell since morning. During her session at BATAE, the director told her that she had unresolved tension in her right arm, shoulder, and left side of her abdomen. I had been so preoccupied with putting the structure in the bedroom, I had barely given a thought to Young-hee's health. Then, as nightfall approached, things grew worse.

"Lie down if you're tired."

I was at a loss as to what to do for her, when Young-hee explained that she needed fresh air again. She also claimed that my actions were only motivated by my own goals and that I was acting selfishly. Then, for a second, I was the miffed one.

"What else can I do? When you call, I immediately come to you, and I stay at your side all day. Today, I went to BATAE and back with you, and built a structure in the bedroom!"

I went a step further.

"Let's hire a caregiver if I'm not any good. Someone you can share a bed with!"

We came out of the apartment under a dark storm cloud of discontent. We did not start talking until we had walked quite a distance.

It was breezy and cool. I thought that Young-hee would enjoy it, but she seemed to be on the verge of tears. Then, she burst out crying.

"You must be getting so annoyed with me! I shouldn't behave like that."

Young-hee sobbed uncontrollably as the cool breeze caressed her cheek.

"How come you're crying? It must be your fatigue."

I stood behind Young-hee and supporting her body against my chest, leaned our torsos back to ease her tension. We also performed stress-relieving exercises as we held hands and faced one another. I dabbed away her tears. I felt sorry.

We walked. After feeling the cooling breeze, we felt a little better.

"Are you planning to hire a caregiver?"

Young-hee questioned me anxiously.

"No, I've been opposed to it from the start. I'll do everything! I'll always be by your side."

Ill, and really with no choice but to rely on me, she was trying to read my thoughts. But oftentimes she seems unaware that she is the patient, and wants to issue instructions and secure confirmations about the most minute details, as if she is at the center of everything. Young-hee must undergo a transformation if she is to ever get out of this mindset . . .

We talked a lot once we got home.

"I promise you that you don't have a terminal illness. It won't kill you. You can get over this ailment with time. There's no denying that you're getting better. Don't be too frustrated if you experience ups and downs for unknown reasons. Your health is getting a lot better. Many others live in considerably worse circumstances than you do."

"Are you positive my health is okay?"

"Sure, that. Whatever the situation, we've always managed to find solutions. So, don't worry! I even built a structure in the bedroom. A crucial breakthrough that will enable us to handle the problem on our own!"

By 11:00 pm, Young-hee was sleeping like a log. (8. 30.)

This Much Today, Farther Tomorrow

WE WOKE UP LATE THIS morning. It was past 10:00 am when we got up. We went for a walk after breakfast, around 11:00 am.

Young-hee's body was more at ease today. As we began our stroll and passed by the adjacent building, she stopped to sit on an outdoor garden stool by the fountain to have a rest.

"Shall we take Banpocheon Trail to the playground today?"

"No, that's too far."

"Let's go as far as the Octagonal Pavilion by the elementary school, then. There's a bench there, where you can rest . . . "

A cool breeze was blowing. We let our feet be our guide.

"My, it's so cool!"

At the Octagonal Pavilion, Young-hee nearly fell asleep. Once we arrived home, she immediately went to bed and took a nice nap from noon until 3:00 pm.

After a late lunch and a quick rest, we went for another walk. We followed the same route we had taken in the morning, stopping at the Community Center where we walked around inside. To leave the building, we took a staircase that went up 37 steps, instead of using the elevator. We got in some nice leg exercise.

At 7:00 pm, we had dinner and watched TV.

"Let's go out again!"

"No, we've already been out twice."

"It's cool outside and you need to digest the food you ate."

Young-hee thought that two outings were plenty.

"All right, let's go! You have to lead me. You're the one who controls my fate."

She then took her medication, and at 8:30 pm, we left the apartment.

It was the opposite of what I remembered from yesterday. I brought along a mat for outdoor use. Taking a reverse course from our morning and afternoon walks, took a path around the apartment complex and stopped at the fountain, where I spread down the mat on the broad stone railing so Young-hee could lie down on it. I covered her body and legs with a long, thin towel and then we repeated our tension-relaxation exercises. It was all very comfy and she almost nodded off. Her body grew calm.

We came home just before 10:00 pm. She fell asleep in no time.

Around 11:10 pm, I went out, walked to the stadium, and came back an hour later.

"Are you back now?"

I promptly sat down next to her and gently exercised her arms and hands.

It was a good day. (8. 31.)

The Lover I Long For, Even When She Is by My Side

"She sat down sometimes, but mostly she listened standing up, and managed the situation flawlessly. Maybe she felt more confident now about having this type of meeting."

Using the Exercise Equipment on Her Own

WE WENT TO BATAE TOGETHER in the morning. She got her diagnosis. Her body has loosened up a lot compared to the earlier exams. When the director instructed her to perform a neck exercise, we heard a "pop" for the first time, which the director deemed to be a good sign. There had never been any indication of improvement in the past, no matter what they tried. Her neck and shoulders were so stiff that she could not feel the massages, and she had trouble turning her neck from side to side. The positive shift has also brightened Young-hee's spirits.

I went to work for the first time in a while, and returned home around 7:00 pm. Immediately after supper, we took a walk. We discussed a number of subjects while lying on the stone railing, including the Joongmin Foundation and Research Institute I dealt with earlier in the day.

Young-hee stated that she wished to go to the Women Professors' Workshop that will be held at our institute in two weeks. It is a wise decision. We returned home after 10:00 pm and she slept well. (9. 2.)

It was already past 11:00 am when we had breakfast. We went for a stroll along the Banpocheon Trail. We continued till we reached the three-way crossroad where we stopped last time. On the way back, we spread out our outdoor mat at the rest spot and did stretches. We did a lot of walking.

When we got closer to home, Young-hee exclaimed that her right arm, which had been stuck at her side and had no feeling in it, was starting to move a little. A strange development! She was over the moon. Might it be a result of our regular walks?

Young-hee fell asleep after lunch. I lay down next to her and as I was drifting off, I felt her cover me with a thin blanket. I woke up to the sound of Young-hee lightly snoring next to me.

Five minutes to five! It was time to leave for church. Young-hee was sleeping in the bedroom, each foot in the handle of a TRX strap and her right hand in the handle of a third strap. It was unlike anything I had ever seen. I believe I now have some insight into Young-hee's innermost feelings. I removed her hands and feet from the straps before I headed to Mass. (9. 8.)

Young-hee went to her doctor's appointment with Prof. Jeon. Her test results were all good. She informed me that the professor had chosen Prof. Ham Bong-jin from the Department of Psychiatry to work jointly with him on her case. Young-hee appeared to be in a cheerful mood, maybe because of the good test results.

I went out for a walk with Young-hee midway down the Banpocheon Trail and back. On the way back, she stretched out on a bench in the park and rested. Walking became very easy.

"Wha—? My right arm!"

At the words, I suddenly looked up to see Young-hee's right arm, which had been stuck at her side, starting to move. Young-hee, however, now complained that her left arm was giving her pain. The right and left halves of her body appeared to be pushing and pulling one another.

She said that she did not feel any strength in her arms. She also revealed that there was a numbness in her hands.

Patients tend to worry about their condition from moment to moment, but their companions are able to see the gradual changes that occur over time. Things are clearly getting better. We decided to face every small obstacle head-on, when it arises. (9. 11.)

A few days before the Korean Harvest Festival, around 9:20 am, I went with my son, his wife, and my grandchildren to the cemetery where my parents are buried. I asked our daughter to go with Young-hee on her morning walk since she could not go to the cemetery with us. Outside, it was a warm day.

Young-hee remarked that at her appointment with Prof. Jeon last Wednesday, she and our daughter-in-law had been kept waiting for over an hour. While waiting, our daughter-in-law began walking with Young-hee, just holding her hand. However, as they walked, Young-hee began to steady herself by placing her hand on our daughter-in-law's shoulder. Even though our daughter-in-law was unaware of it at the time, her shoulder started to hurt the next day. She now understands how much work it takes to walk with Young-hee three times per day. Our son chimed in with a suggestion.

"The problem won't be going away any time soon. Let's hire a caregiver to help out during the day."

Although her condition has much improved, and having a caregiver would make my life simpler, the relationship between Young-hee and the caregiver might create new problems. I promised to talk to Young-hee about it. I advised him to look for a caregiver whom we would be sure to get along with, because in a few days I had to travel to Beijing and Changchun.

Our daughter-in-law interjected that she had already spoken with someone. She asked if we might be able to hire the woman who had come to help her with housekeeping during the holidays. The couple of times we met the woman, she seemed friendly. I felt that she would be fine for the job.

I took Young-hee for a walk in the early evening. We chose a different route today, the new route she had tried in the morning with our daughter. We started from our apartment complex's rear gate that leads to an elementary school. We then decided to move to a quiet area where she could lie down and rest.

This time, I took a band and loosely bound my left hand to Young-hee's right hand. Unexpectedly, Young-hee didn't object. I was happy since it was another important discovery. Coming to our usual rest spot, Young-hee lay down and enjoyed a few nice, relaxing moments.

We went for yet another walk just after dinner. For Young-hee's third walk of the day, we followed the same route as in the afternoon. A full, round harvest moon was high in the sky. I stood behind Young-hee and helped her sway her torso from side to side as I assisted her with her stretches. It seemed like a good exercise. Young-hee enjoyed the sensation of her arms swinging loosely and freely.

We walked with hands banded together—her right and my left—like we had done earlier in the day. Young-hee followed my lead while keeping her right hand totally relaxed. It was a success. An important advance!

When we arrived at the front of the apartment building by ours, we spread the mat out and lay down. The stone railing was cold. I covered Young-hee with her coat and doubled the mat underneath her to prevent the cold air from giving her a chill.

The round moon was directly over us. Young-hee felt better. She shouted at the moon as we made our way back home,

"We're working hard every day!" (9. 13.)

For Words to Be as Beautiful as Flowers

YOUNG-HEE HAD A BATAE APPOINTMENT today. When she came home, I greeted her warmly. Before I could ask her about the session, she informed me,

"The BATAE director told me not to connect our hands with a band when we walk!"

I was quite annoyed by the remark. In fact, just this morning, we had walked for about 30 minutes before she went to BATAE. I would have a lot more free time if we did not go for walks. I could just say "goodbye" as she went out the door. I did it in the hopes that it would help her relax a little more and improve her physical health.

"Sure, it may not be easy, but the goal was to lessen your stress. Isn't it the most comfortable method of walking we've developed? Supporting your arm and wrist as we walk isn't exactly easy, you know, because of your arm pressing downwards. The blood vessels in my wrist nearly burst!

But, we endured all that. We devised a way to help you get the walks you need for the wellbeing of your entire body. What information did you give the BATAE director to cause him to advise against it? How is it possible for him to know what we're doing, and how we're doing it? It's clear from his words that he was listening to what you told him. Did he get the impression that I was acting unreasonably; unilaterally forcing you to do something you don't want to do? If so, fine! I'll play a minimal role! Why must I work so hard? If you don't like it, I'm certainly happy to stop!"

My shattered mood didn't mend easily.

"Words are powerful. Should those be your first words to me after coming back from BATAE? Why do you talk like that, without considering how I might feel? You should learn how to speak! That's the change I want to see! But you stay the same!"

I had lunch and left for work. All I wanted was to get away. I went to work and got a lot done.

After I came home and had dinner, Young-hee and I went for a walk around the apartment building. After getting over the morning's hurt feelings, I apologized for getting angry.

Young-hee said she was to blame. We went to the rest spot in front of the building next door, where she lay down. A round moon was hovering above us. Her body was nowhere close to being relaxed or sleepy. The muscles in her arm were active. When we came home, I assisted her with stretching, and put lotion on her before lulling her softly to sleep. Young-hee's right arm kept jerking uncontrollably.

I tried to ease Young-hee's tension while patiently observing the movements of her right arm. She dozed off for a while. Two hours later, she woke up, and I ushered her to bed and laid her next to me. She still had a small tremor in her right arm. I attempted to relax her arm muscles as I normally do. She fell asleep again after that. (9. 16.)

First Outside Activity and Recuperation

IT WAS AN IMPORTANT DAY today. Colleagues of Young-hee's, a group of female professors, were scheduled to meet in the Joongmin Foundation's seminar room.

We left quickly for BATAE in the morning. I watched them help Young-hee with a new exercise technique. Afterwards, I went straight to work. Young-hee decided to go home first and come to the office after lunch.

Young-hee showed up at 2:00 pm. She enjoyed herself greatly with her coworkers. Young-hee had a radiant smile on her face. The entire time, I stood or sat next to her and gave her whatever assistance I could. We also snapped a group picture. I went around during the conference and took a number of high-res pictures. Young-hee's smile was particularly buoyant. I used Kakao Talk to send one of the images to our son. In response to his mother's display of happiness, he promptly sent back a "thumbs up" emoticon.

The seminar was a huge success. To their delight, her coworkers could see with their own eyes how Young-hee's condition had improved. She felt happier and more confident. She sat down sometimes, but mostly she listened standing up, and managed the situation flawlessly. Maybe she gained more confidence about having this type of meeting.

Her face had been wan and pale like a sick person when her friends last saw her, but today they saw her in full health. It was a joyful event.

When we got home, I got a call from National Health Insurance Service (NHIS). I was advised that I needed to submit a doctor's letter by Thursday if we wished to receive the long-term care service for which we had applied. The social worker asked if everything was going well. I informed her that the hospital had said the patient's condition might not be covered by insurance, because it was a "psychogenic disorder".

According to the social worker, Young-hee was automatically eligible for coverage because the NHIS required medical exams only for patients under 65. A doctor's letter was necessary in order to file the claim, however.

I then attempted to get in touch with Dongguk University Ilsan Hospital to request the letter, and even that proved difficult. Unable to speak with the doctor personally, I was told to sign up for the waiting list in case another patient canceled. The decision would remain pending, because our last office visit was not sufficient proof for the claim. Hampered by hospital red tape!

This evening, I emailed Prof. Park. I stated in my mail that the NHIS had indicated the condition would be covered pending hospital approval, but that if the hospital did not approve it, I would look into alternative options. (9. 18.)

Eun-young, the caregiver, arrived today. She will assist Young-hee while I am away. I had an appointment in the afternoon, so I requested that the delivery of the armchair I ordered, scheduled for later in the day, be moved to an earlier time before lunch. I decided that it would be helpful to show Eun-young how I assist Young-hee, so we asked that she arrive around 11:00 am.

Then, unexpectedly, Dongguk University Ilsan Hospital rang. We had to go pick up the doctor's letter. The patient had to come herself. The institution appeared to have forgotten the rules pertaining to the elderly, which differ from rules for the general patient. However, the prompt reply was appreciated.

Anyhow, she had to go back to Ilsan today. I quickly made contact with Mr. Kim the driver and instructed him to take our daughter and her mother to Ilsan. Meanwhile, the armchair was delivered and placed in a proper spot in the bedroom.

Even though the patient, Young-hee, wasn't present, I used the opportunity to speak to Eun-young about my experiences and warned her about a few safety issues. We all ate together after Young-hee came back, and with Young-hee present, I demonstrated the techniques I had described. (9. 19.)

I left the country on September 20, traveled to Beijing, worked hard there, and came home late in the evening on September 23.

I arrived home around 10:00 pm. I made good time since there was little traffic on the highway at night. How was Young-hee doing, I wondered.

I had made a few calls from Beijing. On the afternoon of the day I left Seoul, Young-hee surprised me by telling me that she had had a 2-hour nap and was watching TV in the new chair. I was chatting with colleagues when I made the call from a wonderful, newly-opened Japanese restaurant in a contemporary-style building in front of Tsinghua University's south entrance. While I was being filled in on Young-hee's encouraging progress over the phone, I thought back on the enjoyable times we had shared with our Chinese colleagues, most notably Zheng Lu.

"Welcome back! I'm sure you did a great job!"

When I arrived at the apartment, Young-hee opened the door and welcomed me. We embraced lovingly like in our youthful days. Young-hee appeared a little disoriented and had a sickly appearance, possibly because she had just gotten out of bed. It was a pitiful sight.

After I washed my hands and came back to the room—before even drinking a glass of water—I tried to help her by tugging gently on her wrists and arms. Strangely, though, her right arm stubbornly remained at her side and wanted to stay there. Young-hee said that her arm was dead as a log. My heart sank.

I took Young-hee into the living room and had her lie down on the Ceragem massage bed, where I helped her stretch her body to relieve her tension. Then, I walked her over to the bed and told her it was time to sleep. We performed a few exercises to get her ready for bed. But the tremor in her right arm was still active and strong. I had her take a pill for the symptom and assisted her with various movements to help her sleep.

Her hands began to feel lighter after a while, and just as in the past, it helped her sleep. Young-hee quickly dozed off. I caught up on everything that needed to be done now that I was home, and I went to bed late. Thankfully, Young-hee stayed asleep and didn't wake up. It was a great relief. (9. 23.)

I spent the entire day at home. The state of Young-hee's health has to be monitored. Eun-young arrived at around 10:00 am. Together, we all went for a walk. Eun-young made every effort to help. I occasionally helped Young-hee with stretching exercises to help her relax.

Eun-young remarked that I look like a pro. Everybody chuckled. Young-hee's arms and shoulders felt better, and her hands soon grew lighter and more relaxed. It was encouraging that she could lift and move her arms on her own.

We took another stroll outside after lunch. While watching Eun-young care for Young-hee, I decided that I should also try to wind down. The situation with Young-hee was significantly different from what I had witnessed the previous evening. She had a softer, lighter appearance. I suggested to Young-hee that she visit a hair salon and get her hair done on the way home from the walk. Young-hee initially agreed, but afterwards stated that she would prefer to take our daughter along because she was unsure which style of straight hair would be best.

When I brought up the matter with my daughter, she recommended going right after supper. Young-hee got her hair done and came home. After the cut, she looked much fresher than before. It had been tiring for her, sitting in the salon chair and keeping her head still, and she motioned that she needed to lie down. I exercised her wrists gently, then lifted her arms above her head and lowered them again, up and down, to release her tension.

Young-hee agreed to take her medication and go for another walk. It was her fourth walk of the day. She was unable to do much. She seemed to be having issues. We put down our outdoor mat and other things on the stone slab at the apartment complex entrance, and I helped Young-hee lie down. Then, we performed a number of tension-relaxation exercises. Young-hee claimed that after lying down, her hip pain subsided. We completed our fourth walk.

By the time we reached home, Young-hee was drowsy. She slept much more soundly in the bed compared to last night. There was no need for further drugs. She took one tablet at 9:00 pm, and by 11:00 she was sound asleep. (9. 24.)

PART 3

...

Relearning Everything

CHAPTER 6

· · ·

*Deep Breaths Instead of Sighs,
Walking Instead of Idling*

Was It This Hard to Breathe?

"He advised me to concentrate on exhaling rather than inhaling when breathing. This would naturally make inhaling easier, he explained. He instructed me to make the "ah" sound, which is akin to exhaling."

BATAE, Unexpected Good Luck

A GLIMMER OF HOPE, PERHAPS? ON the advice of our son, a herbal medicine practitioner visited our home one day when I was experiencing discomfort, cramping, and insomnia. I was unable to leave the apartment and he kindly made a house call.

After hearing about all of my problems, the herbalist asked for my wrist and took my pulse. He then offered to make me a total of forty doses of herbal medicine. He said that it was a concoction of healthy ingredients like deer antler, angelica, and white peony. Taking it didn't produce any instant changes because herbal medicine generally needs time to take effect.

The herbalist, however, also mentioned to our son that he knew someone who provided Chuna Manual Therapy, a form of chiropractic treatment, and that the physician had just arrived in Korea from the U.S. and would be here for a brief period of time. He advised us to go see him, as the physician claimed that conditions like mine could sometimes be treated instantly with a neck adjustment.

I had never heard of Chuna Manual Therapy, and the phrase "pop the neck back into alignment" intimidated me, but I wasn't in a position to go into specifics at the time. My husband suggested that we first find out what it is. He scheduled the appointment and went for a consultation.

After viewing a detailed video of my symptoms, the BATAE director gave his initial assessment:

> "First of all, this doesn't seem to be an issue that should be handled with a technique like spinal correction, though I would need to see the patient in person. Based on the fact that her neck palpitates more on the right side than the left, it appears to be a "psychological" issue, unrelated to the anatomical functioning of the brain, stemming from heightened tension, anxiety, or some sort of fixation. It is possible to prescribe a so-called "customized" approach to strengthen the body's natural powers in response to the patient's condition and needs, as well as a method to relax the tension causing her neck spasms.
>
> Breathing is the best way to relax. Although there are numerous ways to breathe, learning to breathe properly is not easy. Nonetheless, carrying out this task alone can greatly improve the patient's condition. Taking all of this into account, I would suggest a tailored strategy that involves breathing exercises roughly three days a week, which must also be performed at home.
>
> The patient's thoughts, or her sense that she can innately follow her body's flow towards balance, is what

matters most when choosing a treatment strategy, not the feelings of the patient's family members. This must be understood. She must learn physical exercises that encourage relaxation and strengthening, in other words. An excellent way to relax is to have a massage. The impact of strengthening is not produced by massages alone, however.

The patient's "mind" is what matters most. Even while the head appears to be at peace, the heart is rife with conflict. In order to prevent the patient from succumbing to anxiety, depression, or despair, we must support and encourage her with a positive attitude."

In an email to our family members, my husband summarized the contents of the consultation, my condition, and the future steps I might take.

I visited the studio on July 23 together with my husband and son. I had no idea at the time that it was a lifeline that would save me. Its name is BATAE Studio, nearby the Nambu Bus Terminal. The director told us that he worked in the industry for 40 years in the U.S. before recently moving back to Korea. The female trainer working with him is a registered representative. The two co-authored a book called *Sit, Stand, and Walk Properly*, and claimed to be experts in both Chuna Manual Therapy and exercises for controlling the inner ("core") muscles, an important component in treating patients.

BATAE, whose acronym stands for Balance, Awareness, Trust, Attitude, and Efficiency, is "a bodily correction exercise program that restores balance by strengthening weakened muscles and easing stressed muscles, thereby helping patients to maintain flexibility in their properly-aligned joints to achieve and maintain an ideal posture".

I was instructed to lie down on a bed-like device that allows the neck, back, and legs to move independently, and then the director felt my neck. As I lay there, my body was convulsing so violently I was afraid I might fall off the device. Sensing my concern, the director laid a mat on the floor and asked me to lie down on it so he could examine my neck.

Even so, he concluded that a physical examination wasn't possible. The muscles in my neck and back were so tightly knit that he couldn't probe them. He advised me to try breathing exercises instead.

He advised me to concentrate on exhaling rather than inhaling when breathing. This would naturally make inhaling easier, he explained. He instructed me to make the "ah—" sound, which is akin to exhaling. So I walked around slowly, going "ah—".

He advised me to drink water because breathing out and making the sound "ah" while walking can make one thirsty. While I was lying down, the trainer rotated my arm to the left and right, and gave my torso a firm back hug to help me sit up comfortably.

Patients tend to have high expectations for each new treatment method or medication that they encounter. At BATAE, I walked back and forth slowly while breathing for about ten minutes, which seemed like no big deal. After all the aimless walking around, I experienced a feeling of disappointment.

No, expecting an ailment that had developed over decades to be cured in a day or two was greed. I'd have to put a lot of effort into it.

Why My Inner Muscles Were So Tense

Likewise, on the second day, the BATAE practitioners laid a mat on the floor, and began massaging the area below the right side of my stomach, where the inner muscles, or "core muscles", are found. They explained that my inner muscles were tense, causing me to experience symptoms. Using the outer muscles and not exercising the inner ones, had led to my current state. People with tight muscles will typically cry out in pain when pressure is applied to this area, but I didn't feel much of anything at all, which was unusual. Yet, I felt a rope-like sensation in my abdomen when he pressed down on the area to the right of my stomach, and when he seemed to grab the "rope" and hold on, I felt my tremors subside.

I felt much more at ease, even agreeableness, while I lay there, as the director massaged my abdomen and the trainer alternately rotated my right and left arms. After the abdominal check, the director then manually examined the back of my neck. Maybe because the muscles in my neck could now be probed, I was instructed to lie down on a Chuna device known as a "guillotine". He instructed me to say "ah" while keeping my mouth open and sticking out my lower jaw, then warned me not to be alarmed if I heard a "thunk" sound. After placing his hand on my forehead, he turned on the device. He observed a faint movement in my neck. The therapy took about 30 minutes to complete.

The guidance to practice breathing and relaxation techniques at home was crucial. It wasn't easy, but I promised I'd do them whenever I had the chance. My breathing would become erratic as my neck muscles convulsed and hardened, causing me to choke and adding to the stress on those muscles. I felt I had a greater grasp on the necessity of having to relearn how to breathe. Proper breathing wasn't simple.

BATAE instructed me to stop by every day for the following few days. They needed to continue monitoring my condition in order to evaluate whether they could treat my symptoms.

The first week, I went every day. After that, I went three days a week. I eventually started going two days a week.

I felt a sensation of discomfort in early August during a treatment session, while the director was pressing on different parts of my body and gauging my reactions. Although the obstruction had partially cleared, the director said, I was still having problems exhaling. He deemed it a sign of progress that when my core muscles were pressed, I felt more discomfort than I had previously. It gave me a small thrill to hear the praise. It seemed like a window of hope was slowly opening.

Initially, I went to the BATAE Studio with either my husband or my daughter, but from the first week of October, I also sometimes went with my care helper Eun-young and a government-dispatched care worker. I carefully performed the exercises BATAE recommended. Both care helpers and family members paid close attention so they could assist me later at home.

One day, after attending a BATAE session, I noticed a bulging lump on my left elbow. It developed while I was performing vigorous rowing arm exercises. Although it wasn't painful to the touch, it grew larger and larger. Worried, I went to the community hospital. I was instructed to get an ultrasound photo. The doctor advised me to consult an orthopedic specialist, as he wasn't an expert in the field and wasn't sure of the diagnosis. I went to an orthopedic surgeon, ultrasound file in hand.

The orthopedic specialist said that the fluid in the lump could be drained, but leaving it alone wouldn't cause any issues. He advised me to leave it alone. Afterwards, I noticed that the lump disappeared on its own.

When someone is unwell, they're easily made a prisoner of their own anxiety, and a needle can seem like a club. Still, the fact that everything worked out well was a good thing.

My back tremors and neck stiffness were definitely reduced by the medication, but it seems like the BATAE Studio sessions were the most beneficial. I had my first session on July 23, 2019, and went practically every week until February 2020, when the COVID-19 virus grew to pandemic levels and I was unable to leave the apartment. I happened on BATAE purely by chance, but it helped me out a lot. I can honestly say that it rescued me.

The director claimed that he had previously worked with others who had symptoms similar to mine. While most other patients complained of tightness in their lower left inner abdominal muscles, my problem was in my lower right. The director claimed that stress from relationships puts pressure on one's left side while stress from one's job puts pressure on one's right side. I did experience a great deal of stress at work. I recalled that Prof. Jeon had also pointed out stress as the culprit. It was odd though, he said, because I've always been a professor and didn't appear to be under heavier stress than normal.

I'm a quiet person. I often struggled alone and found it difficult to share my struggles with others. I wondered if that might have served as a stressor. I've always had a tendency to be reserved and I watch out for how I come across to others. Perhaps I developed the tendency of keeping things inside as an adult because of the pressure I had to be a "good kid" during my youth.

Walking Again! Thank You, Legs!

"On August 19, my husband, who was constantly monitoring my condition, proposed that we go for a walk together. He was concerned that if I stayed in bed too much, my muscles would deteriorate and I'd eventually run out of energy, which would spell real trouble."

The Little Cheering Squad That Urged Me to Walk

ONCE I BEGAN FEELING PAIN in my inner muscles, I moved on to the next stage of exercise while continuing with the breathing exercises. I was warned by the BATAE director that if I stayed in bed all day and didn't exercise, it would be impossible for me to sit and eventually I wouldn't be able to stand. So, for the first time, I started to practice relaxation methods to release my tension.

Square iron poles are fixed to the BATAE Studio's ceiling, from which are hung exercise tools known as TRX. On August 7, the director instructed me to grab a TRX with both hands and lean forward slowly to loosen up my neck and shoulders. I was able to follow his directions with the trainer's assistance, and the exercise was quite helpful.

In fact, my husband had always been supportive of muscle exercises and had emphasized to me repeatedly that I should do them.

"The patient's responsibility is typically to take the medication the doctor prescribes. But if the patient takes

173

the medication and just stays in bed all the time, the patient will continue to be a patient indefinitely. The patient may become unable to stand due to weight loss and the concurrent decline in muscle mass caused by the uncontrollable muscle activity, making daily life difficult. Things are thrown out of balance when this state of affairs persists. What happens when one day, owing to a small mistake, the patient slips and falls?

Yet one still wants to stay in bed, since that is what is easiest at the moment. When compelled to go outside, one can manage without too much trouble. There is a powerful desire to adapt. But, as soon as one gets home, one immediately settles for comfort. How can the patient get past this? That is the big challenge."

I was loaned a TRX by the BATAE Studio and instructed to test it out at home.

When he got home, my husband hung the exercise tool on the door of the study across from the bedroom. He secured it by closing the door. I put the techniques I'd learned at BATAE into practice. My husband's first suggestion was to have our daughter order me a TRX of my own.

Unfortunately, at home, I couldn't do the exercises like I did at BATAE. To hang the TRX properly, iron bars have to be mounted vertically, allowing the straps to hang down like a net. Later, Mr. Kim, who is skilled in such things, bought the supplies and installed an approximate structure in our bedroom.

The bedroom was soon transformed into a BATAE workout area. I was now able to exercise my arms and legs at home. Despite the fact that we were unable to fix an iron bar horizontally below the ceiling like they did at the studio, I was able to lie down more comfortably when I put my wrists and ankles in the handles and allowed my hands and feet to hang suspended in the air.

My mood was improving, though I didn't express it to my husband much, and I was more determined than ever to put the work into doing my exercises. I believe that this served as a trigger for my "model student syndrome"—a chronic condition characterized by the need to perform every task flawlessly, diligently, and precisely.

Maybe the heat was to blame for my rapidly declining energy. Except for when I visited BATAE studio, I spent the entire day lying in my bedroom with the A/C on and my limbs hanging from the rubber straps hanging down from the iron bars. When my grandchildren came to visit, though, my gloomy and depressed thoughts were carried away like the wind.

"Wow, Grandma's room has a swing!"

"Yeah, weird! I wanna play on it!"

The grandchildren first mistook the strange apparatus installed in the bedroom for a piece of playground equipment. Once they realized it was a tool to speed up my recovery, they tried their best to help me with my exercises. They used their little hands to pat at my limbs, or knead and massage them.

When the grandchildren visited us with our son, they would sometimes lie down next to me and join us as we practiced meditation. Or, when my son and I were on the mat that was put out on the floor, they would watch from the bed. They complained that it was cold in my room because the A/C was set so high. Shivering, they would climb into bed and hide under the blankets, pretending to meditate for a few moments before dozing off.

While meditating, I noticed when I opened my eyes that they were unable to remain still, tossing and turning, or lying upside-down on the bed and staring down at me. When our eyes met, they started giggling. I then felt a lot better.

How could playing with their ailing grandmother have been fun for the kids? Maybe they made a "deal" with their mom that if they kept me entertained, she would let them play video games later. Youngsters are normally like that. What could I do, given that they were the number one contributors to my happiness?

That's how I survived the challenging summer.

I Walked Outside and Met the Breeze

MY HUSBAND VISITED PROF. PARK on August 2 to discuss an urgent matter. I was having a hard time managing life day-to-day. Even with the A/C on, it was hot, and I sweat a lot. I was constantly lying down and had trouble falling asleep at night. But after attending BATAE Studio for a while, I could tell that things were gradually getting better, so I started going on walks with help from my family. Yet, I was still confined to a bed for much of the time, and I found it a difficult habit to break.

On August 19, my husband, who was constantly monitoring my condition, proposed that we go for a walk together. He was concerned that if I stayed in bed too much, my muscles would deteriorate and I'd eventually run out of energy, which would spell real trouble. We started off taking walks with his hands almost completely supporting mine. How fortunate I was to be able to do this—to leave and explore—that was what I thought.

The first few walks were restricted to our apartment building. Our building is on somewhat higher ground than the other buildings in the same complex, and when leaving the building, one can view a cozy, round front yard garden by the walkway. *Maehwa* (apricot), peach, and other fruit trees, as well as perennials like lilies, day lilies, asters, and silver grass, spring up between irregularly shaped rocks in the garden, ensuring that lovely flowers bloom all year long.

At the garden, one can see a narrow trail moving off, flanked by a lot of maple trees. Walking there is great. When the maple leaves change color, the trail is a beautiful sight with a motley array of red, yellow, and green leaves. In the spring, the air is perfumed with blooming lilacs. From there, one can descend a short flight of wooden steps, and beyond that, one comes to a fork in the trail where it is deliciously cool when the wind blows. At least it was when we went there in the evening. My husband and I typically went out at night.

"Ah, the coolness!"

"It's nice, isn't it?"

"Absolutely. I believe I'll get through this."

I opened my arms as widely as I could and just took the refreshing breeze into my lungs. The heat made every day a struggle, but when I went there, where it was so cool, I felt like

I could handle anything that came my way. The crisp air must have lifted the heavy, sorrowful sensation from my heart and increased my determination to get well again. Even though my body felt heavy and I wanted to stay in bed, the memory of that "sweet wind" gave me the willpower to stand back up.

As one descends the wooden stairs, a pond can be seen ahead to the left and to the right. Directly ahead, there is a cafe with a cloud-shaped roof. Outside, round tables and chairs are set up with large red parasols that open out to block the sun. The pond's little fountains spouting cool water give it a unique feel. The spot is always busy with people because of its nice atmosphere.

After passing the pond and turning right, one comes to a small winding path and a small arching bridge. After crossing the bridge and turning left, you come to a spacious lawn with a tall zelkova tree that stands as the apartment complex's "guardian". The tree was transplanted there ten years ago when the apartments were constructed. Since then, it is said to have just barely survived. On the stately lawn sit three large, handsomely-shaped rocks. The scene, barren of water, has an atmosphere reminiscent of Kyoto's Ryouanji Garden. The main difference is that there is green grass instead of sand.

Turning right from there brings one to a small-scale model of "Manmulsang", the famous view in the Geumgang Mountains. Despite their small size, the pointed rocks, cascades, and pine trees work in unison to mimic the Geumgang Mountains in North Korea. Continuing along, if you turn right and cross the street, you come to a slope that leads up to a higher level of ground. This slope was hard for me to climb. I always had to warm up first, bracing myself for the challenge and taking deep breaths as I went up it.

I was always winded after reaching the top, as though I'd scaled a mountain. Yet I was also happy. I felt as though I'd accomplished a great feat. We would then proceed along for a short distance until we came to the fountain in front of the adjacent building, our final stop.

On the fountain's stone railing, my husband would stretch out a large towel he had prepared, help me lie down, and assist me in performing exercises like rotating my arms and raising them above my head. Though he sometimes took me there during the day, he usually took me at night. Until September 20, when Eun-young came to take care of me, he took me for walks on practically a daily basis.

I exercised every night, walking with my husband and lying on the railing while gazing up at the moon and stars in the sky. Before my illness, I had only gazed at the moon once a year when making a wish on the Lunar New Year, but now I saw it each night.

The new full moon always appeared out of nowhere—it seemed the last one had appeared just a few days before. Perhaps "time really does fly", or perhaps, strangely enough, when you see the moon every night, the new moon appears before your memory of the previous one has faded.

I wondered how many full moons I'd see until I was healed. Thanks to my illness, I began to glance up at the moon, though it hardly interested me before.

How About Muscle-Strengthening Exercises?

"Can I walk that far?", "Sure. You can handle it. We'll go slowly."

I Tried a Medicine Called 'Walking' . . .

I N FACT, I'D TUCKER OUT, soaked in perspiration, just from walking around the grounds of our apartment building. I'd lose energy even when I stopped to rest periodically throughout the walks. I wasn't aware of how much stronger I was becoming from the continuous walking.

I first started walking just around the apartment complex, for about a month. I then progressively increased my distance. My legs were alright, but my upper body—neck, shoulders, arms, hands, and back—was shaking, in pain, and susceptible to paralysis. Walking was no problem as long as someone held my hand.

It strikes me now that I have been exercising consistently since I was a child. I played tennis practically every evening during the summer I was a 20-year-old student in the U.S. That habit of exercise allowed me to sail through the first stressful years of my professorship after returning to Korea. After that, I would hike on the mountain near our apartment, take in the fresh air, and go for walks on the weekends and whenever I had free time.

Even when my husband and I traveled to Aix-en-Provence for an EU project, I kept up my fitness routine. One day, en route to Sainte-Victoire Mountain, I happened upon the Stadium Georges-Carcassonne sports complex. I jogged around on one of the athletic fields there. The location was excellent: a sprawling park with large grassy areas and a large river next to it. There were several soccer fields, an American football field, huge indoor and outdoor swimming pools, basketball courts, table tennis courts, and numerous other sporting facilities. Because the nicer turfed grounds seemed to be for parties who reserved in advance, we availed ourselves of a small, unturfed sports field.

I recalled being advised to avoid putting too much stress on my knees as I grew older, so I began limiting myself to just walks. I noticed, however, when I turned and looked around, that I was the only one walking. In reality, all the older people were running. I shortened my stride and began doing light running exercise.

It was next to impossible to escape the sweltering sun because there was only one large tree in the area. No matter how lightly I ran, I always sweat bullets. Sometimes, when I changed directions and ran southward, a bracing breeze from Provence known as the "Mistral" would blast over my perspiring body and cool it.

I felt content and refreshed after finishing my run and lay down for a while on the grass beside the sports field. The feeling was like being in Heaven. Despite the fact that it was quite a distance from downtown, I went to the grounds and ran and ran for good stretches of time, I so liked the cool, refreshing feeling after exercising. My health greatly benefited from all of the brisk walking and jogging I did under the hot Mediterranean sun.

My former residence in Bangbae-dong was located behind Mt. U-myeon. I liked to hike there whenever I had the opportunity. Although close to a main road, it felt like I was trekking deep in the mountains. I felt as though I was in another world, the scenery was so breathtaking. There are three hiking trails at Mt. U-myeon: the high, medium, and low trails. At the time, I could manage all three, but I think they'd all be challenging for me now. The Banpocheon Trail and a sports complex are a stone's throw from the apartment I live in now, and all the pathways are level and suitable for walking. All of this meant that until I got sick, I could keep up a regular walking routine in my spare time.

I am grateful for my legs. Even when I was sick, I had no real difficulty walking, my legs are strong. My hand just needed to be held by someone. My arm felt like I was lugging a barbell. After a while, I started taking longer walks outside of the apartment complex, along a pathway that stretched about 100 meters long.

"Can I walk that far?"

"Sure. You can handle it. We'll go slowly."

Although I had it in my head that I could pull it off, the first time I tried, it took some mettle. I worried that should I need to stop midway through the walk, I might end up stuck and stranded. What would happen then? My husband took my hand and reassured me that everything would be fine.

I gave the trail the moniker "Dawn Redwood Trail" since it's lined on both sides by tall dawn redwoods. It's mostly level, with the exception of one daunting uphill stretch, making it overall an excellent route for walking.

The trail was enjoyable during the daytime because of the lovely surroundings, but it was no less enjoyable at night when the street lights came on and illuminated it, making it as bright as day. It was a pleasant walk any time of day or night. The uphill part was challenging at first, but it grew easier with time.

I went for walks with Eun-young or the government care helper when my husband wasn't around. At these times, the person with me always held my hand to support me. Without the helping hand, I couldn't walk very far. During the walks, I would do arm rotations, take sit-down breaks, and perform arm-pulling exercises to loosen up my shoulder muscles. I always had a water bottle so I could hydrate myself.

Learning New Exercises and a New Way to Walk

EVERY TIME I VISITED BATAE Studio, the instructors had me relax my inner muscles and do the specified order of rowing exercises, which I performed diligently and carefully. They gradually made me do different exercises once I showed some improvement, no doubt resulting from my consistent practice.

I once learned a new exercise that involved sitting down and standing back up while having my hands held for support. It was a squat-like exercise, and at first it wasn't easy to do. I had no strength in my arms or shoulders and my back hurt and my legs shook. Because I had trouble moving my body, they instructed me to grip the straps of a TRX hanging from the ceiling, and pull on them to loosen up the muscles in my shoulders. Even that would have been impossible to do alone, without someone supporting me. I also set up a TRX at home and used it there. But things didn't go so well.

The next exercise I performed was to stand with my arms raised against a wall and perform small vertical push-ups. BATAE assured me that doing this would relax the muscles in my shoulders. I was told to do the exercises at home, and I tried my hardest to comply, but it was difficult to do them at home as well as I did at BATAE. When no one else was using the elevator, I would stand facing the corner, put my hands on the wall, and do vertical press-ups, leaning in and pushing back out.

From time to time, I tried doing a few repetitions. My body initially refused to move because my shoulder muscles were stiff and knotted up. As time passed, I was gradually able to move in and out, pushing and pulling, as my shoulders began to stretch out and loosen a little.

I learned several exercises, and then I learned how to walk. I walked by leaning slightly forward while getting supportive pushes from behind. The director warned me that after the first five steps, I would start to slouch. Although it wasn't easy, I followed his instructions. My right shoulder hiked up a little when I walked, and my arm movements were awkward and unnatural.

I was reminded once more of Prof. Jeon's suggestion that "you have to relearn everything from scratch". From breathing to walking, I had to essentially relearn everything.

I put a lot of work into relearning how to walk and doing the other exercises up until February 2020, when I was no longer able to attend BATAE due to the Corona outbreak. Yet, others would still tell me that my gait appeared abnormal.

The Armchair I Bought Because Sitting Was Difficult

"I had it for about two months and didn't use it much, but one day I sat in it and before I knew it, I fell asleep. I slept a good two hours. The chair started to feel more comfortable after that, and I eventually warmed to it."

Escape from the Floor— the Beginning of Life in a Chair

I VISITED PROF. PARK IN ILSAN on September 17. On the way home, I spotted a row of furniture stores. Since I couldn't sit upright for long in a regular chair, the task was to get a chair that was comfortable enough for me to sit in. Since we had stumbled onto these furniture stores by chance, my husband decided to look for an armchair that would meet my needs.

I didn't know what kind of chair to get or which brands were popular because I wasn't usually interested in armchairs. Unsure of where to go at first, we entered a furniture store that looked like it had been in business for a long time. After explaining my condition to the proprietor, my husband asked him which chair would be most suitable. He showed us both floors, downstairs and upstairs, and suggested a few different models. I tried out a few of them and chose the one that was the most comfortable—a reclining armchair.

When the chair arrived a few days later, we put it in the bedroom. My son had brought me a new tiny TV, which my husband set up so that I could watch it from the chair in comfort. While sitting in an armchair was more comfortable than regular chairs, it wasn't as cozy as lying down, and I still spent a lot of time in bed.

I had it for about two months and didn't use it much, but one day I sat in it and before I knew it, I fell asleep. I slept a good two hours. The chair started to feel more comfortable after that, and I eventually warmed to it. This meant that without my knowledge, my body was gradually getting better. From then on, I often sat in the armchair, watched TV, and napped. I eventually broke my habit of lying on the floor.

The armchair was responsible for an unforeseen development: My feet were washed nightly. My husband sat me down in the chair and bathed them in warm water. It helped me sleep much better when he did this. It wasn't a matter of just once or twice. My husband washed my feet every night for about two years before his own health suffered a downturn, at which point he could no longer do it. Amazing husband! Once I fell ill, he was determined to do anything he could for me. I asked him several times not to, but he still did it. Flinching, I told him that even Jesus washed His disciples' feet just once . . .

He would pour warm water into a large basin, have me stick my feet in, heat extra water in an electric kettle, set it aside, and then stoop down to wash them. As the water started to cool, he would repeat the process by adding more warm water from the electric kettle.

I felt bad for my husband crouching on the floor and washing my feet. I pleaded with him to stop, but he insisted. He was relentless, like he wanted to make me his queen. Although it was pleasant, I found it unsettling, and I argued with him about it every night. Be that as it may, I could sleep better because of his efforts.

One day, my son bought me a Ceragem massage bed with the expectation that it would relieve my fatigue.

I was unable to use it at first, since I didn't understand how it worked. Then later, a serviceman came and showed me how to operate the control functions. I discovered how to vary the vibration intensity, temperature, and other settings depending on my specific health issue, such as cold, indigestion, or back pain. I've used it a lot since then. If I slightly increase the temperature on the 'massage' feature, the marbles moving back and forth under the mat make my back toasty warm. I've mainly used the 'strengthen immunity' setting.

I already owned a massage chair that my son had bought for me. I couldn't use it when I was first diagnosed, when I had muscle spasms. The first time I tried to sit in it, the massage seemed to make my already stiff muscles contract even more, and it hurt a lot. I screamed and leaped out of the chair. It took a long time after that for me to submit myself to another chair massage.

I liked the Ceragem bed because I could lie down and it didn't make my muscles tense up too much. So my husband took the massage chair, and I used the Ceragem to relax. Ceragems and massage chairs each have their unique advantages. When you've finished your meal and are ready to unwind, the massage chair is ideal, and the Ceragem is good after your food has digested.

The massage chair's vibrations are powerful and quickly refresh you. Ceragem slowly warms you up while massaging your back (ideal for a quiet environment with music playing softly in the background) so I would fall asleep almost instantly after lying down on it. Both the chair and the bed were very helpful once the tremors stopped. I've been very satisfied!

Gift of Herbal Medicine, Wrapped in My Daughter-in-Law's Filial Piety

I T WAS TOWARD THE END of September. One day, my daughter-in-law mentioned to me that one of her former classmates from elementary school was a pharmacist who had also studied traditional herbal medicine. He traveled all the way to Seoul to see me from Cheonan, where he lived. He carefully asked information about my health, took notes, and by and by prepared some herbal medicine for me that he shipped to my home.

There were five different types of medicinal ingredient: cattle gallstones, polysaccharide extract, a natural sedative, a granulated plant extract, and traditional medicinal boluses. According to the book *The Principles and Practices of Eastern Medicine*, the sedative solution improves symptoms developing from the psyche; polysaccharide extract, all natural, prevents dryness in living organisms; and cattle gallstones increase energy and replenish the blood. The boluses provide quick relief from spasms, stiffness, and numbness.

I prepared the herbs by combining the first three ingredients in a large cup, then dissolving the granules in some hot water and combining it with the other ingredients. Then, after waiting for 10 to 30 minutes, I took the boluses, washing them down with the herbal concoction. I had to wait 10 to 30 minutes to allow for the natural fermentation of the dietary fiber, sea salt, and fermenting bacteria in the granules, thereby enhancing the absorption rate and the medicinal impact.

I began taking the herbs on September 27, and happily, the numbness in my fingers gradually began to disappear, perhaps as a result of the medicine's effects.

Midway through May 2020, after taking the medicine for seven to eight months, the Cheonan pharmacist contacted me again. He asked me to describe my present symptoms, took notes, and after a day or two, a new packet of medicines arrived.

This time, there were five medicines: traditional herbal pills; a blue decoction; a red decoction; AugustMed Octacosanol; and traditional medicinal boluses. The traditional herbal pills are purported to relax the mind and promote sleep, the blue decoction is good for making clogged blood interact with the meridian system, the red decoction improves physical constitution and restores cells in the skin, muscles, blood vessels, and nerves to their normal state, and Octacosanol boosts muscle strength and endurance. The boluses were identical to those in the first packet.

At first, I experienced problems like diarrhea and frequent urination, but over time, the diarrhea went away and the frequency of my urination decreased. I continued taking the medicines for almost four months before stopping. My Western medicine-trained doctors didn't approve of me utilizing natural medicines. During my checks, they told me that certain tests revealed liver enzyme levels that were higher than normal.

There were also funny moments. My son and his wife came to me one day in late June 2019 holding two unusual white jars. Because I had always been so healthy before, they were very worried about my sudden illness.

"What are those? Are they jars of honey?"

"No, Mom. Some people recommended this."

After filling each jar halfway with salt and then adding water to the salt, they placed one in our bedroom and one in the study.

When I questioned what they were doing, they explained that they had been quite concerned and had approached someone who had advised them to try this, on the suggestion that our apartment, particularly the areas my husband and I use as our bedroom and study, might have bad *qi* energy. The absurdity of the idea aside, I couldn't help but chuckle at the thought that if the jars ever broke, our rooms would be a sea of salt water. I enjoyed a good laugh with my family.

Everyone believed that any idea was worth a try because of how terribly my condition was deteriorating. I was grateful to my loved ones who cared about me, regardless of whether the jars worked or not. We were in a difficult situation at the time and were desperate.

The First Reinforcement—A Care Helper!

WALKING AND SITTING BECAME DIFFICULT in September of 2019. I had to purchase a walking aid.

Our driver, Mr. Kim, informed us that Gu-eui-dong has a huge medical supply warehouse where they have everything under the sun. Large hospitals only have one or two different models of walker in their medical supply stores. Mr. Kim suggested that since I'd be the one using it, I should go choose it myself. Despite the fact that it wasn't easy in my condition, my husband and I went to the supply warehouse.

I looked around and chose two walkers—one for indoor and one for outdoor use. I purchased the simplest and least expensive one to use indoors. I also picked out a large rubber exercise band to suspend from the iron bar structure set up in our bedroom.

As I was about to pay at the register, the cashier asked me if I received long-term healthcare services. My husband and I were unaware of such services, so we asked him for more details.

The cashier handed me an application form and said that I'd probably be eligible. He stated that we could apply right there, inside the store. On the spot, my husband completed the paperwork, which was then faxed to the NHIS. Then we forgot about it.

My husband had to travel to Beijing for a conference on critical sociology. He was anxious about leaving me alone. He had to be in Beijing; there was no way to cancel the trip or arrange for a substitute. I needed someone to look after me during his absence. We hired Eun-young, whom my daughter-in-law knew well and whom I'd previously met several times. A single woman in her

40s, Eun-young had a slender frame and appeared frail, but she was kind-hearted. Before my husband left the country, he spared no pains explaining to her what a caretaker he had been for me.

Eun-young began working for us around the end of September. Just like my husband and daughter, she cleaned my face and applied body lotion. She helped me get dressed, go to bed, and perform exercises like arm rotations after my shower. She served me food when I was hungry while I stood clinging to my walker. She also gave me my medications on time.

Whenever we went for a walk, she brought along a big towel and a water bottle in her backpack. When we reached the fountain where my husband and I frequently stopped following our walks, she stretched out a towel on the railing for me to lie down on, and then assisted me in stretching out my arms, just like my husband did. All of the exercises were ones I had learned at BATAE Studio.

She gripped both of my hands in hers while we walked and carried nearly the entire weight of my right arm. She'd sometimes face me and hold my hands from that position, or she'd walk beside me, my right arm in her right hand and my left arm in her left hand. It must have been taxing for her to carry my right arm, which was as heavy as a barbell, while walking at the same time. When I asked her if it was difficult, she replied, "Ma'am, the harder it is for me, the more comfortable it is for you", She reassured me that she could handle it. Her heart was like an angel's.

CHAPTER 7

. . .

The Small World I Began to See While Walking

You're Getting Better, It's Nothing to Be Ashamed Of

"Every morning and afternoon, someone came to walk with me, exercise with me, and help me eat, and so a rhythm began to build."

Strategy for Recruiting a Care Worker

AFTER A SERIES OF TWISTS and turns, the long-term care application faxed from the medical supply store was approved, and in the end, I was allowed to access elderly long-term care insurance services. The NHIS called us to make arrangements for guardian education in preparation for receiving long-term care. My daughter visited their office, went through guardian training, and was given a certificate. Later, after looking up a few long-term insurance care facilities, we got in touch with one that had an A rating.

A few days later, a social worker and a prospective care worker visited our residence, along with the center's director. That day, Eun-young was helping me exercise by rotating my arm as I lay on the floor. In that state, I went through an interview for a care worker assignment.

I qualified for three hours of care work per day. Because we would have to pay out-of-pocket to get more hours, I drew up a timetable that allocated time between Eun-young and the new caregiver.

We decided that Eun-young would mainly visit in the afternoons and the care provider in the mornings.

The day the care worker arrived, we returned to the Gu-eui-dong medical supply center and purchased a higher-quality indoor walker. It was really comfortable to stand and lean forward on it because the front handle was rounded and soft. Its wheels also rolled very smoothly. It was somewhat pricey, but because long-term care insurance partially covered it, I was able to get it for 15% of the original cost.

I had a great time using the new walker. I could move around indoors much more comfortably and with less effort. I also leaned against it when I ate from the tray set on the dining table. It was far more manageable eating that way than trying to sit on a chair.

Unfortunately, after working for two days, the care provider announced that she wouldn't be able to continue. She said she had also informed the center's director. She found it too tiring to support my arm as I moved about, and it was too difficult for her to exercise with me. There were a few times when the care worker unintentionally let my hand slip from her grasp while we were doing the squat exercise. I cautioned her to hold on firmly in case I should fall backward and suffer a concussion. That seemed to irk her. The caregiver said that she was too old and weak to continue, that she could no longer do what the job required. Naturally, she said that she would wait until a new caregiver came to take her place.

I was introduced to a new candidate by the center's director. On that day as well, Eun-young was rotating my arm as I lay on the floor. After seeing me in my state, they left, and a few days later the center notified me that the new candidate would also be unable to do the job.

Until that point, I didn't realize that the caregivers were avoiding me. I made the decision that the next time a candidate came, I shouldn't be lying down, and I tidied myself up to appear less sick.

It seemed that the center's director was having some trouble finding a caregiver. Thankfully, the third care worker applicant took the job and stayed with me.

Then, my husband traveled to Jilin University in Changchun, China for an academic conference. The conference, honoring the eminent Chinese philosopher Gao Qinghai, couldn't be postponed or cancelled. The university, moreover, wished to hire my husband as a chaired professor for five years. Because he was to give a lecture at Yanbian University after the conference, his travel schedule would be longer than a week. My husband's concerns grew as his scheduled absence grew lengthier.

While my husband was away in China on business, our son joined me in the evenings to help me with my walking and exercises. Given that I'm short and my son is tall, it was physically awkward for both of us when he held my right arm as we walked. After a week of walking together, my son told me that he had a sore hip joint and could no longer help me with my exercise. He's a very kind son, and imagining the suffering he must have endured, I couldn't help but feel sorry for him.

In fact, after months of supporting my right arm during our walks, my husband's left arm finally gave out, too. He was unable to raise or extend his arm freely due to excruciating pain in his left shoulder. I'm sincerely sorry to think that I've caused hurt to my family. My right arm was so heavy, and everyone suffered terribly.

Strange People Singing, Dancing, and Walking

THE CAREGIVER AND EUN-YOUNG MADE it a high priority to attend BATAE Studio to learn how to perform the exercises. This was necessary so that they could comprehend the types of exercises I performed there, pick up the new ones, and follow along with me every day at home. So once a week, we all went to BATAE Studio together.

They learned muscle-relaxing techniques like squats, where I sat down and the care worker stood holding my hands and helped me stand up and sit back down. This helped relieve the tension in my arm, neck, and shoulder. They also learned how to rotate my shoulders, and received tips on how to help me walk correctly. The care provider visited on Mondays and Tuesdays for the entire day as well as on Wednesdays, Thursdays, and Fridays in the early morning. Eun-young came to take care of me on Wednesday, Thursday, and Friday afternoons, as well as on Saturdays. On our evening strolls around the apartment complex, my husband would have me lie down on the fountain railing and rotate and tug on my arms to exercise and strengthen them.

By doing these things, I was able to gradually achieve stability in my daily life. Every morning and afternoon, someone came to walk with me, exercise with me, and help me eat, and so a rhythm began to build.

My recovery from illness was greatly aided by the ordered lifestyle that started with the care worker and Eun-young showing up at the scheduled times. My physical condition gradually improved, and I noticed that my mental energy level was increasing. Surprisingly, though, I continued to lose weight—I weighed 10 kg less than before. My face had lost fullness to the point where I had double eyelids, which I'd never had before, and I could see that my limbs were now skinny.

I spent my days walking my customary route around our apartment complex, with its blossoming flowers and lush trees, with the care worker or Eun-young supporting my right barbell arm, exactly like my husband and my family did.

The caregiver and I would get winded during the circular course, and stop several times before we reached the top of the slope. When we arrived at our destination, an empty bench near the fountain, she would lay me down on a big towel and help me do exercises like rotating my arm.

Passers-by would sometimes comment:

"Are you in pain, ma'am?"

"Do you need to go to the hospital?"

"Who are those women, mommy? Why do they do that?"

Other people would stare at us curiously, as we often held hands or exercised on the bench. Even perfect strangers approached us and asked what we were doing. Children would ask their mother questions about us. We must have looked odd, even to them.

Adults naturally wondered why people were singing and dancing hand-in-hand in broad daylight. It would look 'weird' to anyone who wasn't aware of the circumstances.

People on the street stared at us as we danced around mimicking a traditional dance as the two of us clasped hands and sang songs like *Arirang* following the technique we learned at BATAE Studio. Some busybodies remarked, "It'll be more entertaining if you play a cassette tape!" or "Don't hold hands while you walk!"

Once, as I lay on the bench and performed my arm rotation exercise, someone cried out, "Don't lay the baby there!" from an upper story of the apartment building. I was lying there rotating my arm when someone saw me and gave a chef's kiss: "Primo technique!"

When I first heard these comments from neighbors and onlookers, I felt embarrassed and ashamed, but as I reminded myself that it was a form of treatment that was making my body better, I determined not to let it bother me. I choose to ignore it and focus exclusively on my training regimen.

There were quite a few songs we sang while we walked and exercised. From slow songs like *Arirang* or *Doraji Taryeong* to fast ones like *Milyang Arirang*, *Dal Taryeong*, and *Arirang Mokdong*, we went through a lot of classics and ditties. When Eun-young mentioned a song she knew, we looked up the lyrics online and sang it boisterously. One beautiful song I'd never heard of is called *A 100-Year Life* (*Baekse Insaeng*). The lines were absolutely relatable to me:

> *When I'm 60 and the other world comes to get me /*
> *Tell 'em I can't go because I'm still young*
> *When I'm 70 and the other world comes to get me /*
> *Tell 'em I've still got work to do*

When I'm 80 and the other world comes to get me /
  Tell 'em I can't go because I'm still needed here
When I'm 90 and the other world comes to get me /
  Tell 'em I'll go on my own, so don't rush me
When I'm 100 and the other world comes to get me /
  Tell 'em I'm going to pick a good time and a good day
Arirang Arirang Arariyo / Going over the Arirang
  Hill again
When I'm 80 and the other world comes to get me /
  Tell 'em I can't go because it hurts my pride
When I'm 90 and the other world comes to get me /
  Tell 'em I'll go on my own, so why are they here again
When I'm 100 and the other world comes to get me /
  Tell 'em I'm looking to the day I'll be reborn in paradise
When the other world comes to get me up at age 150 /
  Tell 'em I'm already in paradise now
Arirang Arirang Arariyo / Stay healthy, everyone!

While singing the song, I thought to myself, "I'm not old enough for the next world". And with that, I stepped up the intensity of my exercise.

My Right Arm Now Lifts Easily

"My right arm, which had been as heavy as a barbell, miraculously lifted upward after a few weeks of acupuncture. Moreover, the cost of the treatment was only 1,000 won, about $1."

The Effects of New Prescription Drugs and Acupuncture

MET PROF. HAM BONG-JIN FROM the Department of Psychiatry for the first time on November 13. I was a little bothered that it was a psychiatry department rather than neurology, but we gave him a thorough account of my symptoms, the course of my treatment, the exercises I did at the BATAE Studio, and the medications I'd taken. The doctor didn't seem particularly friendly, and he spoke in a rather serious tone—possibly because Prof. Jeon had specifically asked him to help us.

When I received the prescriptions and opened the pill packets, I noticed that the Alpram and Rivotril were the same, but that Sensibal, an antidepressant, had been substituted for Lexapro. On December 11, a brand-new medication called Neurontin Capsules—used to treat epilepsy or seizures—was prescribed. Like Rivotril, it appeared to be a fairly potent drug. Also, Prof. Ham urged me to only receive treatment at one hospital since it would be inconvenient to visit two facilities for the same illness.

My husband and I both felt that it was a good idea. On November 19, my husband emailed Prof. Park to express his gratitude for the care I had received from her and to let her know that Prof. Jeon had asked Prof. Ham to treat me.

I'm not sure if it was the additional things I did, like exercising at BATAE and regular walking, or if the new doctor's medication was unusually potent and worked well for me, but after meeting the new doctor, my symptoms seemed to dramatically improve. At long last!

In the meantime, someone recommended that I visit an excellent oriental medicine clinic well-known for acupuncture. The person suggested I try it after we learned that my inpatient examinations revealed no issues. Since May, she had been urging me to visit the clinic, but I kept putting it off because I believed my Western-medicine doctors would be more competent. I scheduled an appointment with her and went for an acupuncture session at the end of the year. I was frightened of needles, but that couldn't be helped.

The clinic is close to the Sinsa subway station. My husband and I went with the person who suggested the treatment. The clinic provided therapeutic acupuncture as well as traditional acupuncture. I informed them that my right shoulder hurt. I was instructed to lie face down during the procedure. I had to remain in that position for 15 minutes after the insertion of the needles. Because I couldn't endure the discomfort, the session was ended after 8 minutes. They said that in the future they would have me lie on my side, and thereafter I was treated in that position.

My right arm, which had been as heavy as a barbell, miraculously lifted upward after a few weeks of acupuncture. Moreover, the cost of the treatment was only 1,000 won, about $1. As a result, I began to stop by the acupuncture clinic on my way home from BATAE.

I was aware of acupuncture's significance in Asian medicine, but I had no idea it would have such a profound impact. The therapeutic acupuncture at the clinic was also quite beneficial.

However, as my right arm regained its motility, my left arm, which had been numb and cold after a period of feeling weak, began giving me problems.

Heaven gives with one hand and takes away with the other . . .

Hope is the Heart of the Flower, the Heart of the Person

"Then, in my heart, I imagined myself encouraging her, urging her to take one more step. These were all things I had missed before falling ill."

Our Front Yard Garden and *Maewha* Blossoms in the Snow

OBSERVED THINGS I'D NEVER NOTICED before once I started going for walks. Every tree in the apartment building looked so graceful and lovely. Tiny flowers beckoned me to gaze at them—flowers I'd never noticed before.

Hmm, hmm, hmm. I lifted my face, focused my nose, and followed the scents. It was spring and I was just noticing it. In the front garden of our apartment building in the spring—no, even before spring had arrived—the most tenacious flowers were the *maewha* or apricot blossoms.

It was February, and pink blossoms had begun to open on the little *maehwa* tree, whose branches drooped instead of poking skyward. Little *maehwa* buds had impulsively peeked out. How trying the previous winter must have been! The tree was completely covered in snow, creating "a *maehwa* in the snow" like in old oriental paintings. How gorgeous!

I quietly drew nearer. Then, all of a sudden, I came to a stop and fell into a moment of solemnity. The tiny flower buds, which had turned crimson in the cold like a baby's cheeks, had melted the snow. The scarlet beauty of the *maehwa* blooms were fighting a hard battle against the frozen snow, and they were giving it everything they had.

More *maewha* blossoms began to bloom after the pink ones. The most fragrant were the plain white. The grounds of the apartment complex host many such *maewha* trees, and I was pleased with their appearance and lovely, refreshing scents in the spring. After the petals fell, leaves emerged on the trees and before long, fruit hung in profusion from their branches.

Forsythia is the flower that signals spring's arrival. Cherry and forsythia trees grow in abundance along the Picheondeuk Trail in Banpocheon. After spending the whole winter looking at dark gloomy trees devoid of leaves or blossoms, I was overjoyed to one day suddenly find a forsythia twig with yellow blossoms poking out from the February grey. Every time I went for a walk, I looked carefully to spot new golden buds, to see how they were coming along. Then, when the spring cold hit and the buds froze and dropped from the branches, I was fretful at the sight.

Pink water lilies, too, began to bloom on the pond. These lilies, a common sight throughout the summer, not only have a lovely color, but also a graceful, smart appearance that refreshes the eyes.

Even the fountains at the Cloud Cafe, with their multiple water effects, appeared more refreshing than before. The force of the gushing water as it jets into the air and the splash with which it plummets into the pond, were exhilarating. In the past, I would have thought it all loud and noisy.

I was now more aware of the mallard ducks waddling around the pond. I spent a lot of time studying them. I discovered for the first time that the pond is home to red, white, and yellow-colored koi. I occasionally saw some terrapins clambering up a rock and basking in the sun. Maybe they were turtles.

Under trees, between rocks, and hidden beneath large flowers, little flowerlets and grasses with unknown names were glorying to the fullest during their brief existence of a few days on this earth. Birdsong could also be heard when it was quiet.

All of these new discoveries gave me happiness and joy.

Support for Our Sick Neighbors and Me

MY RECOVERY WAS GREATLY HELPED by the meticulously designed and properly tended garden in front of our apartment building. The most splendid and beautiful season is spring, when all types of flowers are in bloom. In fact, I'd been going through life oblivious to and unappreciative of this beauty my whole life. Every spring and summer since moving into our present apartment, I had traveled to France, so I was unaware of how gorgeous our apartment's—no, our country's—spring was. The phrase "How could I not have known!" perfectly captures my state of mind at the time.

The autumn leaves, as well as the spring flowers, were now even more breathtakingly beautiful. A lot of baby maple trees were planted along the walkway through the front garden. Towards the end of October and beginning of November, not just one color, but a variety of red, yellow, orange, and green leaves harmonized together to create a picturesque landscape.

When the trail is covered with leaves in late October, the atmosphere becomes seasonally richer. After getting sick, I started going for daily walks and observed an array of new things and sights. I gained a fresh sense of awe for beauty. It seemed as though I was only now becoming aware and appreciative of the full moon.

While I was healthy, I was unaware of others' illnesses, but now that we were "birds of a feather", I became conscious of my sick neighbors. On my morning walks, I observed people enjoying the morning breeze from their wheelchair, pushed around by someone, as well as people hobbling around with walkers.

I focused on one pair in particular. Every morning, the husband wheeled his wife to the Cloud Cafe near the pond where they shared a cup of coffee. While her husband devotedly went to order the coffee and bring it outside, his wife would patiently wait there, her head lowered with her hat on. They showed up every morning, without fail. I was in awe of the husband's tremendous devotion and concern for her.

Another person I frequently saw was an elderly man, wheelchair-bound, accompanied by a female caregiver who appeared to be in her early 50s and who was constantly with him. I had a quick chat with her. She said that she'd been his care assistant for almost two years. She added that because the man disliked being hurried, she had to do everything slowly to avoid upsetting him; otherwise he would lose his temper.

"Don't hold hands!" the gentleman growled when he spotted my caregiver holding my hand as we walked. "Get up!" he said when he spotted me lying down on the bench. This, despite the fact that he himself was in a wheelchair. He presumably was giving me advice out of nostalgia for what he missed doing.

A short-haired woman who appeared to be in her twenties, or perhaps teens, was also a regular. She could walk only with great difficulty. She clung tenaciously to her walker while receiving support from behind by a helper. She struggled with her steps as she stumbled along precariously. My heart sank as she approached the bottom of the stairway.

I saw her trembling as she made her way up the three or four steps with help from her caregiver. The realization that I had been in her shoes brought tears to my eyes.

Then, in my heart, I imagined myself encouraging her, urging her to take one more step.

These were all things I had missed before falling ill.

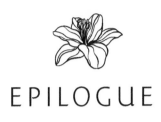

EPILOGUE

. . .

The Basis For Turning This Case of FMD Syndrome Into a Narrative

As we conclude this book, my wife and I would like to share the following thoughts while COVID-19 and its mutations rage. As much as science has developed, has the world become clearer to us? Can one say that life will be safer as modern medicine progresses forward? No one can say "yes" with confidence. The more one knows, the more one does not know. It is a paradox, yet it is true. The more scientific development has progressed, the greater the level of mankind's reflection on uncertainty has grown. When a vaccine is developed, the virus proceeds to challenge us again with ever more virulent mutations. Medical knowledge and technology cure diseases, but on the other hand, new, inexplicable diseases arise and cause new frustrations. Functional Movement Disorder Syndrome is one such example.

We can see from looking around that even among younger generations, a significant percentage of people suffer from symptoms for which the precise nature of the disease is unknown. Following countless medical examinations and experiments, it seems that there is nothing wrong with the patient, yet the patient's body is in pain. These are situations where a structural cause cannot be identified, yet the body is still not functioning properly.

This story about FMD Syndrome was turned into a book because of our desire to describe, in a simple way, the patient's confusion as she experienced symptoms of an ambiguous origin, her relief at finding a small escape route after much searching, the disease's shifting patterns, and the value of family support when the patient found it difficult to manage the healing process on her own. It is not a description of a patient finding the cause of her illness and treating it using tried-and-true medications alone. It charts a process of trial and error, carried out in total darkness, of diagnosing the ailment and developing a treatment strategy.

The first significant confusion on the journey was the use of prescription depression medication while experiencing a strong tremor in the neck muscles. Honestly, it was difficult to accept the argument that the horrible involuntary movements of her body were signs of a mental illness. Furthermore, while taking the medications, she seemed to get worse. So, in the era of free and open conversation, the family began searching for a courageous doctor. *How about this physician? What about that specialist?* Each of us looked far and wide before settling on a health recovery strategy that we felt was most effective. There was nothing wrong with that, insofar as everyone genuinely wanted to help the patient.

But the environment surrounding the disease became perplexing and contrary to what we had hoped, and over time, our anxiety and fears only grew worse.

I made a choice at that moment: No! Taking a detour wasted time and was exhausting. The condition will not get better if you do not trust the doctor. The family's job is not to provide medical knowledge or information. Instead of leaving it to the doctor, the family's job is to comfort the patient so that the anxiety and fear do not grow in her heart; to talk about good memories and the bright future ahead; and to do our best to alleviate any inconveniences in the patient's day-to-day life. I resolved to my wife: "I will put everything else to the side and do my best for you, so follow me." In this way, we were able to maintain some sort of order in our home.

This book may be found useful for its breakdown of FMD Syndrome and its extensive descriptions, through experience, of how our body and mind work in tandem. Naturally, not all of this functions in the same direction. There can be a vicious cycle where the muscles experience tremor, causing the mind to grow anxious, in turn causing the muscles to grow more agitated. Alternatively, there can be a virtuous cycle where the mind is stable and the tremor commensurately decreases, in turn providing comfort to the mind. When she went to the doctor or performed something that was scheduled in advance, she did not concentrate on her muscle spasms because her thoughts were elsewhere. Walking outside and breathing in the cool wind can cause a cascade of events to occur throughout the whole body, cheering the heart and reducing feelings of heaviness. In this manner, the bodily and mental processes can interact, the direction of which can fluctuate depending on the circumstances.

We know from experience that when stress builds up and accumulates in the mind, it might manifest itself in a form that is not a mental illness, even though an exact causal relationship may not be understood. It might result in physical dysfunction, such as quaking muscles, stone-hard shoulders, and an arm that won't move from one spot and stays stuck by one's side. The ability to trust one's doctor is crucial for treating this condition, yet taking the recommended prescriptions is alone insufficient. A family that can lovingly embrace the anxiety and terror that the patient feels internally is a 'must' for managing FMD Syndrome. This message is contained in our book.

My wife, who is the main author, wrote the prologue, therefore I decided to write the epilogue as her co-author and caregiver. Above all, I hope that this book, which is a story, will be helpful to patients and families experiencing related symptoms. If it does, that will be our greatest joy and reward.

May 2023
Han Sang-jin

ABOUT THE AUTHORS
AND THE TRANSLATOR
. . .

About the Authors

Shim Young-hee was born in Andong, North Gyeongsang Province located in the southeastern part of Korea, and graduated from Gyeongbuk Girls' High School before entering the Department of English Literature at Seoul National University (SNU).

Han Sang-jin was born in Imsil, North Jeolla Province located in the southwestern part of Korea, where he graduated from Jeonju High School before entering the Department of Sociology at SNU.

When the two entered the graduate program of the Department of Sociology at SNU in 1970, they began dating, crossing the social barriers that existed between the southeastern and southwestern provinces of South Korea at the time. They became much closer while going through a period of 'campus turmoil' in 1971, when Han was unjustly arrested. The pair got married after Han was acquitted and freed from police custody. The pair then left for Southern Illinois University in the United States, where Shim obtained her doctorate in critical criminology in 1978, and Han obtained his doctorate in 1979 specializing in Foucault's and Habermas' theories. There, they had one son and one daughter.

Shim returned to Korea first. While she was at Jeonnam National University, she witnessed the horrors of the Gwangju Uprising. In deep shock, she went to Germany and joined her husband, then a postdoctoral researcher at Bielefeld University, and the two pursued their research endeavors in Germany and England.

Then, while teaching at Hanyang University, Shim was dispatched to the Korean Institute of Criminology in 1989 to conduct a nation-wide victimization survey on sexual violence and sexual harassment, a first for Korea. This, along with her researches on issues such as gender equality and the elimination of domestic violence and sexual violence, helped establish the foundation for a national women's legislative movement in the 1990s. Against this background, she has since served as the president of the Korean Association of Women's Studies, as a co-representative of the organization Women Making Peace, and as chair of the Women's Committee for the Peaceful Unification Advisory Council. She is currently an emeritus professor at Hanyang University and an executive director of the Joongmin Foundation, a public interest corporation.

Han, while at SNU, took an active part in transformational debates, advocating a 'Joongmin theory' amidst confrontation between the two extremes of military dictatorship and popular revolution. At the counsel of Kim Dae-jung, founder of the First Opposition Party competing in the 1988 general election, Han rose to leadership of the Presidential Committee for Policy Planning. He has served as the President of the Academy of Korean Studies, and is currently an emeritus professor at SNU and chairman of the Joongmin Foundation.

• • •

About the Translator

Ga Baek-lim studies Korean literature and has translated a number of Korean short stories and longer books. He is currently a research fellow in Seoul.

Milton Keynes UK
Ingram Content Group UK Ltd.
UKHW041923310823
427823UK00001B/49